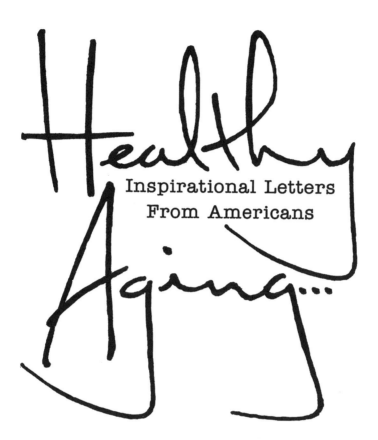

Healthy Aging

Inspirational Letters
From Americans

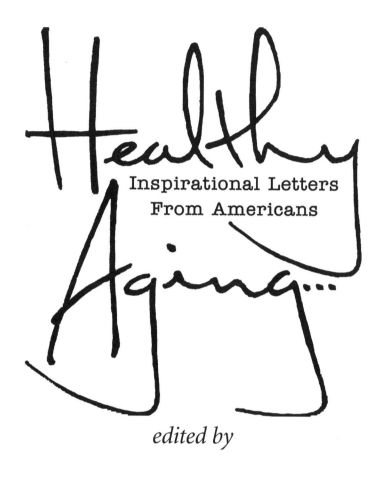

Inspirational Letters
From Americans

edited by

Carolyn E. Worthington

Thomas J. Dryden

David M. Chauner

Rutledge Books, Inc.

Bethel, CT

Rutledge Books, Inc.
8 F.J. Clarke Circle, Bethel, CT 06801

Manufactured in the United States of America

Cataloging in Publication Data
Healthy Aging : inspirational letters from Americans /
    edited by Carolyn E. Worthington, Thomas J. Dryden and
    David M. Chauner
      p. cm.
    ISBN 1-887750-54-1
      1. Aging—United States. 2. Longevity. 3. Aged—United
States—Attitudes. 4. Middle aged persons—United States—
Attitudes. I. Worthington, Carolyn E. II. Dryden, Thomas J.
III. Chauner, David M.
    305.26--dc21   97-65754
                                                CIP

Acknowledgments

This book could not be possible without the thousands of people who entered the national letter-writing contest we conducted as part of our national Healthy Aging™ Campaign and in celebration of Healthy Aging Month in September. First and foremost, we would like to thank them.

We would also like to thank the United States Postal Service for sponsoring this contest, and the people there, who knew the value in promoting the one franchise the Postal Service has that no other organization or business can touch — the ability to deliver a personal letter, inexpensively, in a short amount of time, to virtually any mailbox in America. In these days of faxes, e-mail, and phone calls, there is still nothing more gratefully received or cherished longer than a personal letter.

Thanks, too, to the marketing and communications people at Postal Service headquarters in Washington who helped us most directly with this project: Loren Smith, Sid Shulins, Robin Minard, Larry Dingman, Monica Hand, and Fem Lucero. We also want to thank the thousands of Postmasters and postal employees around the country who eagerly went out into their communities to promote the contest and demonstrate that the local Post Office cares about the people it serves.

To encourage entries and to promote the value of writing, we produced a "Write From the Heart" writing kit which was used by many community groups to conduct writing workshops. We want to thank our partners in this effort, The National Council on the Aging and specifically its president, Jim Firman, and its program manager, Bobbi Johnson, who worked hard to shape the kit and oversee its distribution.

There are many other national health and aging organizations and professionals who provided support and encouragement to the Healthy Aging Campaign and to the letter-writing contest including the U.S. Administration on Aging (Fernando Torres-Gil, Carol Crecy, Irma Tetzloff, and Priscilla Jones), National Association of State Units on Aging (Jim Whaley), National Association of Area Agencies on Aging (Janice Fiegener), AARP (Carol Cober), National Postal Museum (Jim Bruns), Elders Share the Arts (Susan Perlstein and Susan Willerman), Southwestern Connecticut Agency on Aging (Edith Serke and Christine Lewis), and Dr. William Evans.

We thank those who spent hours publicizing the contest to local aging organizations and post offices including Harrison Edwards Public Relations (Carolyn Mandelker, Candice Fitts, and Bonni Kogan) and Lorraine Abelow Public Relations (Lorraine Abelow and Fred Ianotti). And a special thank you in this area goes to our national spokesperson and cultural icon, Willard Scott who, in one short day, proved that Healthy Aging is a gift of caring, positive attitude, and good humor.

A final, special thank you goes to our honorary judges who not only carefully read their selections but came back with some incredible insights and observations of their own which we are proud to be able to share with you: Jane Brody, Dr. Robert Butler, Dr. James Birren, Art Linkletter, and Dr. Ida Davidoff.

Dozens of people were involved in launching the letter-writing contest and seeing it through to its successful completion, the culmination of which is the publication of this book. In particular, we would like to single out and thank Judy Dryden and Ruby See for their help in screening entries during the preliminary stages; Michael W. Noomé for his superb design and illustrations which grace this book; Steven Badalamenti, Cynthia Detuzzi, Ben Dryden, Stuart Dryden, Linda Lopriore, Inger Mirabile, Elenita Morris, David Randall, and Maria Zanghetti for counting words; and Denise Toth, Dan Bartlett, and Aronette Clayton for their superb administrative services which kept us organized under an avalanche of mail. Thanks also to our hard-working administrative assistant, Diane Monaco. And to the following who, in many untold ways, supported our efforts: Timothy, Michael, and Helen Chauner, John and Kay Worthington, TC, and Sweet William.

The Editors
Carolyn E. Worthington
Thomas J. Dryden
David M. Chauner

CONTENTS

Introduction

Aging, from our baby boomer perspective, is a reality that has only recently begun to emerge from the shadows. We've hardly adjusted to being adults and parents, let alone started to think of ourselves as growing old ... or even middle aged. But, as we are more and more inclined to admit, the future is now, and how we handle growing older has become very important. Suddenly its not "where will I be in five years?" its "how will I spend the next fifty?"

This prompts some interesting questions: Do we have to accept physical decline? Will we be able to afford a quality lifestyle if we live to be "elderly?" How will our interests, activities, and passions change? What about our attitude? How will we adjust?

These kinds of questions, and encouragement from a few key people, first led Carolyn to explore the concept of what older people can do, not what conventional wisdom suggested was no longer possible with advancing age. The result was her public television special entitled "Our Nation's Health...Healthy Aging®."

It was an eye-opener. Women pumping iron in their 90s. A men's baseball team you could only join if you were over 75. Older people playing, volunteering, taking singing lessons. People who, in unexpected ways and settings were admittedly happier, healthier, and more relaxed than at any other time in their lives. It became apparent that there was a world of positive, upbeat older adult role models behind the headlines. Old age wasn't necessarily a haven of disease, decline, loneliness, and irrelevance.

And so the Healthy Aging Campaign was launched ... a national initiative to focus attention on the positive aspects of growing older. It was a turning point not only in our corporate goals, but in personal ones as well. Carolyn explains:

After interviewing hundreds of specialists in the aging field, profiling many "pioneers of aging" and spending hours in the editing room studying their comments and lifestyles, both my corporate and personal life were changed forever. Perhaps it was native American, John Pino, who began walking for exercise in his 80s around his pueblo in New Mexico and then, in his 90s, went on to compete in the Senior Games, that made me begin to think about the myths of aging. Or was it Rose Karsh, who began to lift weights in her 90s and was finally able to walk unassisted by increasing her muscle mass, that made me join the Y, start pumping iron and walking on a daily basis? Or was it Ida Davidoff, 93-year-old practicing family therapist who lives independently and told me "You don't grow old, you become old by not growing" that sparked me to begin taking piano lessons and appreciate every waking moment as a special point in time? I was inspired and excited.

It was Dr. Robert Butler who perhaps helped us most to shape the principles of our Healthy Aging Campaign. Through his work with countless older Americans, he had discovered a common thread among those who aged well. First, it was a positive attitude ... a sense of purpose in life. And he believed that the path to successful aging was marked with road signs: physical, social, mental, and financial. When we found people in whom these aspects of life have come together, he said, we would find those who define the spirit of Healthy Aging.

We wanted to explore this. We thought it would be interesting to meet more self-fulfilled older people and to somehow get them to tell us, in their own words, what Healthy Aging meant. And better yet, why not let other Americans benefit from their discoveries, particularly those of us who are coming up from behind and perhaps thinking about this for the first time.

And so we decided on our mission for the first Healthy Aging Campaign ...

Through the development of public/private partnerships and the magic of cause-oriented marketing, companies interested in reaching the expanding "senior market" chipped in to help fund and spread the Healthy Aging message. And who better to deliver that message than the United States Postal Service?

Thanks to them, we were able to encourage thousands and thousands of older Americans from all across the country to write letters to us ... to future generations ... to you ... about the real meaning of Healthy Aging.

Tom got very passionate about this. He organized the national letter-writing contest and helped establish necessary contest rules so we could publish a manageable number of entries*. He read every letter that met the judging criteria (it took three months!). And he made some interesting observations:

As members of the fitness-obsessed baby boomer generation ourselves, Dave, Carolyn, and I had some preconceived notions about the nature of the advice we would receive, particularly since the assignment was to draw upon personal experience to inspire future generations to improve their physical, mental, or social health.

Frankly, we had expected that a substantial percentage of entrants would share tips for fat-free diets or their own personal exercise regimens.

We were wrong.

Overwhelmingly, the vast majority of entrants wrote not about physical fitness, but about the importance of mental fitness. Specifically, they wrote about the importance of maintaining a positive outlook, finding strength within themselves to meet life's challenges, including aging, head-on.

So, if you're one of those millions of baby boomers who are convinced that a firm, trim body is the single most important thing you need to age healthily, there's a key lesson to be learned from reading this book.

Sure, the hours you spend at the gym, and the effort you make to eat right, will help you age healthily.

---

* This book represents only a small portion of the letters we received. The winning entries from each age category (50-59, 60-69, 70-79, 80-89, and 90+) from each state and the District of Columbia have been included. Each letter was judged according to contest rules: 200 words or less, aptness of entry to Healthy Aging theme (40%), inspirational nature of advice to future generations (30%), and originality (30%).

Ultimately, however, it's a positive mental attitude that will see you, and us, through our golden years. Based on the responses we received, an active body isn't as important as an active mind, or a positive attitude.

While each entry was unique, we found that many of our entrants focused on the same basic themes. In no particular order, here are some of the most common tips for Healthy Aging our entrants shared:

See the World/Expand Your Mind: *After a lifetime of raising children and working, older Americans love to travel—to see new things, and experience new cultures. Many entrants cited the Elderhostel program, which enables them to visit far-flung destinations on a budget while enjoying adventures in learning.*

Watch Game Shows: *Dozens of entrants advised future generations to watch* Jeopardy! *to keep their minds razor-sharp. (Interestingly enough, only one entrant claimed to find mental stimulation in* Wheel of Fortune. *Take that, Vanna!)*

Laugh Loud, Laugh Often: *A good sense of humor is essential. Many entrants told us they start the day off on a light note by reading the comic sections of their local newspapers. (Those over 60 tended to refer to the comics as the "funnies.")*

Eat Your Fruits and Veggies: *Mother's advice way back when was right. Our entrants eat them now. They ate them growing up.*

Give of Yourself: *We were awed by the altruism of our writers, who are overwhelmingly generous with the most important thing they own—their time. They volunteer for everything from the Peace Corps, to visiting local nursing homes, to teaching youngsters to swim.*

Choose Your Parents Wisely: *Repeatedly, entrants cited members of their own families who had lived to be 90 or older, and attributed their own longevity to their genetic inheritance.*

Seek Inspiration: *Hundreds of entrants began or ended their letters with quotes that have shaped their own philosophies on Healthy Aging. At least 100 entrants cited the following, by Robert Browning:*

> *Grow old along with me!*
> *The best is yet to be...*

Keep the Faith: *Belief in a higher power is of paramount importance, especially among those in their 50s and early 60s. Interestingly, the older the writer, the less likely he or she was to mention faith.*

God Bless America: *Many, many respondents expressed their gratitude to be living in the United States, where one has choices, as a key to Healthy Aging.*

Walk, Walk, Walk: *You don't have to be a triathlete (though we received plenty of entries from those) to stay fit. The #1 most-often-cited physical activity was walking.*

Go for the Gold: *We received many entries—even in the 90+ category—from people who have participated in the Senior Olympics program, on both local and national levels.*

Be a Beauty Queen: *An astonishing number of women told us they enjoy competing in beauty pageants, such as the Ms. Senior America program.*

If You're a Man, Get Married: *Interestingly enough, many married men attributed their longevity to the loving care and companionship of their wives. Women, on the other hand, didn't claim their husbands helped them live longer.*

A Penny at a Time: *Hundreds advised future generations to set aside a percentage of each and every paycheck...and to forget about it.*

Look to Mentors: *Never underestimate the importance of setting a good example. Hundreds of entrants cited mentors who set living examples for Healthy Aging, especially parents and grandparents.*

Lastly, we were impressed by the ability of entrants to express themselves in writing. Generally, the quality of writing—handwriting, spelling, sentence structure—was superb. Is the ability to express oneself in writing something that comes with age? Or is it true that younger Americans aren't taught to write as their elders were?

As you will see from the introduction to each section of the book, picking the final winning letter from each age category from every state was not easy. We wanted to publish many more letters than we could and we wanted to personally thank everyone who tried to pour his or her soul onto a blank piece of paper, whether or not they made the final cut.

We accomplished our mission and more. We discovered that age does not have to be feared. We learned that people want and need to communicate vital thoughts and ideas as long as they live. We found that wisdom and piece of mind truly belongs to those who have traveled far, observed much, and want to keep going.

But most of all, we had an unusual opportunity to look through a window to the future, our future, and through that, realize that life is what you make of it, no matter what your age or situation happens to be.

In summary, we would like to raise a toast to 100-year-old Helen Quackenbush of California (who admitted she still enjoys a good martini), and to the more than 6,000 other 50+ Americans who took the time to enter the contest. Though only a small percentage of entries appear in this volume, you're all winners in our book.

So sit back, read the best of the best, and reap the rewards of the nearly 500,000 years of collective experience shared by our letter-writers.

As we were, you'll be inspired.

The Editors
Carolyn E. Worthington
Thomas J. Dryden
David M. Chauner

About the Editors

Carolyn E. Worthington is a communications professional, television producer, and founder of Educational Television Network, Inc., a non-profit company in Wilton, CT which specializes in creating award-winning programs for public television, principally in the areas of health and aging. Most recently she created the Healthy Aging™ Campaign and has become recognized among health and aging professionals as an authority on quality-of-life for aging Americans.

Thomas J. Dryden is president and executive creative director of Dryden And Petisi Promotion, LLC., an award-winning sales promotion agency in Westport, CT. He is responsible for structuring the Healthy Aging letter-writing contest, and as a professional writer, establishing the criteria by which the entries were judged. His fascination with the subject resulted in him personally reading, over a three month period, every entry received.

David M. Chauner is chairman of Educational Television, Inc., a marketing specialist, entrepreneur, and writer. As a journalist, his byline has appeared in *The New York Times*, *Sports Illustrated*, and numerous other national and regional publications. He is the principal author of *The Tour de France Complete Book of Cycling* (Villard Books, 1990) and a two-time Olympic cyclist who lives by the spirit of the letters ... never give up!

For information on quantity purchase of this book and a complete list of additional Healthy Aging™ Campaign materials, videos, and discussion guides, please send a #10 size self-addressed stamped envelope to:

ETNET
P.O. Box 7536, Dept. BL
Wilton, CT 06897-7536

WINNING LETTERS FROM THE 50-59 AGE CATEGORY

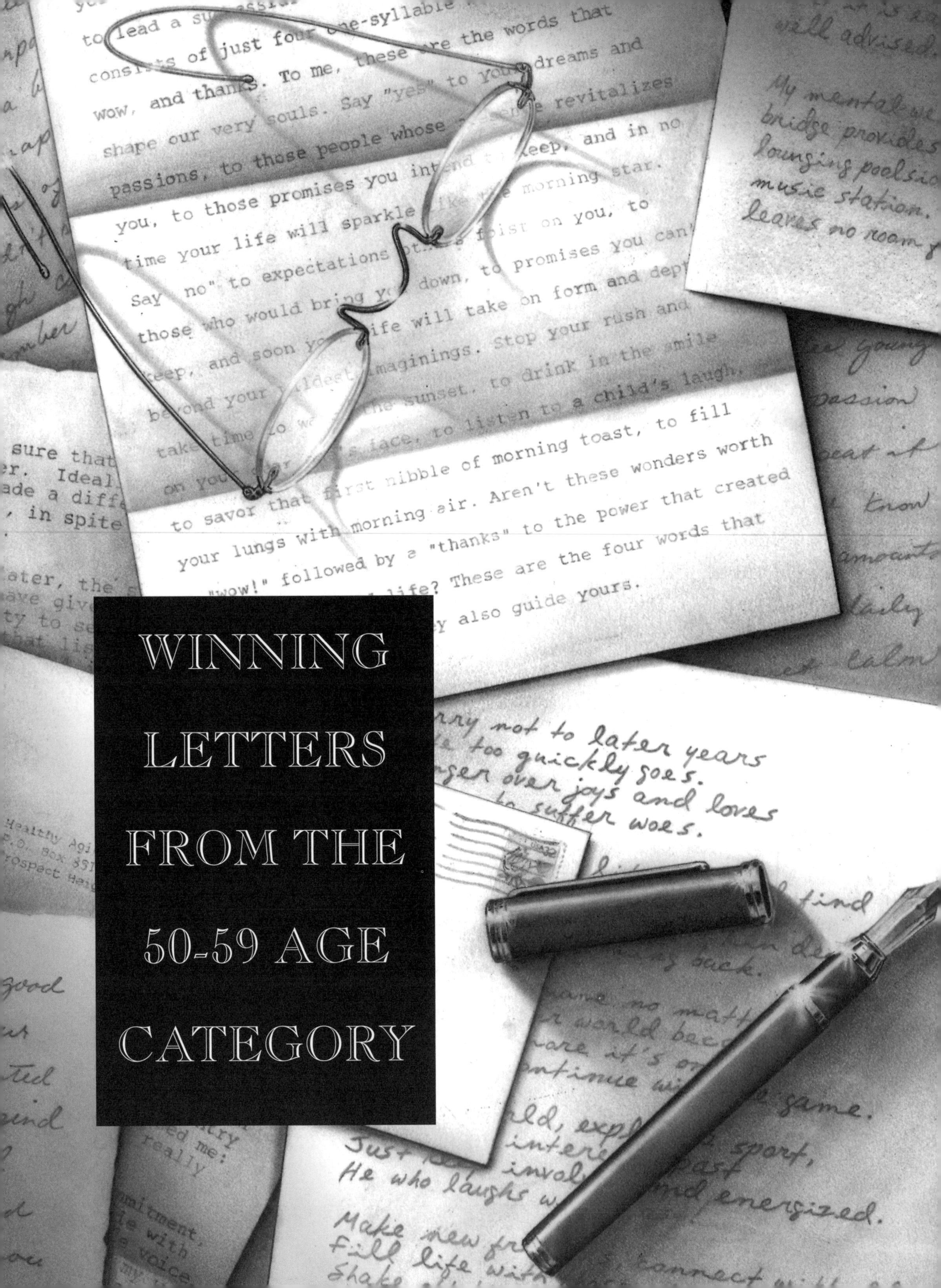

Jane E. Brody

JANE E. BRODY is a science writer and the Personal Health columnist for *The New York Times*. She was born on May 19, 1941, in Brooklyn, New York, where she still resides with her husband, Richard Engquist, and their 11-year-old mixed-breed spaniel, Max. Their twin sons Erik and Lorin, are both married and living independently—and healthfully—sharing their mother's interest in a good diet and regular physical exercise. Ms. Brody majored in biochemistry at the New York State College of Agriculture and Life Sciences at Cornell University and holds a master's degree in science writing from the University of Wisconsin. After a two-year stint as a general assignment reporter for *The Minneapolis Tribune*, in 1965 she joined *The Times* as a specialist in medicine and biology and created the Personal Health column in 1976. She is the author of nine books, including three best sellers: *Jane Brody's Nutrition Book*, *Jane Brody's Good Food Book*, and *Jane Brody's Good Food Gourmet*.

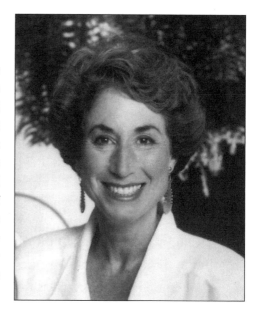

STATE OF MIND

Healthy Aging is not an act of God or a lucky throw of the dice. Healthy Aging is a state of mind—an attitude—and a willingness to resist what appears to be the easy way out. As these letters so clearly show, those who are aging healthfully have not necessarily led charmed lives. Many have suffered horrid tragedies. They have lost children or spouses long before their time, lost jobs unfairly, failed at business, lived in poverty, worked unconscionably long hours, carried the burden of two or more people, suffered debilitating illness, etc. Yet they have learned secrets of successful living that have enabled them, not just to carry on, but to be useful to friends, neighbors, total strangers. They have learned that living solely for oneself and inside oneself is the route to disappointment and depression, but they have also learned the limits of what they can give and still have something left for themselves. And they have learned that a smile is the best umbrella to protect them from the slings and arrows of outrageous fortune.

When I was 19 years old, a very wise, grandfatherly professor at my college convinced me to put my philosophy of life down on paper. What I wrote then has guided my life since. I wrote that when life ends, I should be able to write my own epitaph, a celebration of what my life has meant. My mother had died two years earlier, at the tender age of 49, having worked as an elementary school teacher since age 17 and having just one vacation with my father unaccompanied by her two children. No one was happier than I to reach and pass the age of 50. I learned from my mother's too-early death that one cannot, should not, must not postpone life, that each day must be lived as if it could be your last, that life is a perpetual exchange of give and take and that a balance must be maintained between the two. I learned to take the time to smell the roses, watch the birds, enjoy the sunrise. And most important, I learned to share my time and talents with others.

In my middle age, I am not without sorrows or pain or disappointments. But I continue to see life as a glass half full, and I continue to try to fill the other half. That, to me, is Healthy Aging.

ALABAMA

Sharon Y. Reed
Age 59
Sheffield, AL

Healthy Aging is a sign of the time we live in. To the caveman it meant simply survival, but to the aging 50 and over crowd of today, Healthy Aging has taken on a whole new meaning. The 21st century is rapidly becoming a reality and it demands to be lived and experienced to the fullest. Age 50 is no longer old and neither is 90. They are just numbers applied to mankind's identity with self. There is so much more I can do at age 59 that I didn't even think of doing when I was younger.

My mental health speaks volumes and allows me to continue my growth of knowing me, no matter what age I am. My physical, social, and financial health do not crumble with age because they are supported and standing upright on a solid foundation built with good, sound mental concrete. *I am ageless while aging.* Good mental health has made it so.

The 21st century will dance with us, the elderly, and we will, in turn, dance with the 21st century. With good mental health we can see ourselves as we really are, *wondrous human beings at any age.*

ALASKA

Steve Adams
Age 56
Fairbanks, AK

Healthy Aging is a simple, yet difficult process, with the key word to success being r-e-s-p-o-n-s-i-b-i-l-i-t-y.

Accepting responsibility for your health, education, and overall welfare is essential. Life is a precious gift, Healthy Aging is the result of the successes of your responsible actions.

Society is not responsible for you, your lifestyle, or your success or failure on what can be a long and difficult road through life. Most of the road will be uphill and you will find the helping hand you need at the end of your own arm, not some kind of a "gift" from the government.

You are what you are because of the decisions you make, not the "breaks" you get, the status and/or background of your parents, the neighborhood in which you grow up, or your monetary value.

Good eating habits, avoidance of substances and "friends" that can harm you, the proper amount of rest and exercise and a good mental attitude are all your responsibility, and contribute immeasurably to Healthy Aging. Emphasis today often seems to be placed on failures, but look around, there are success stories from all corners of this great land to inspire you. Accept responsibility for your life today!

ARIZONA

Curtiss F. Barker, II
Age 57
Scottsdale, AZ

Dear Americans:

Healthy is as healthy does.

Use humor as a key to Healthy Aging. Us it to unlock your past, present, and future experiences.

You will always find a chuckle looking back—your first date, school, the Big Game, your drill instructor, work, marriage, kids. A large part of your memory will be humor. It's healthy.

Humor is not so easy to find in the present because you are serious about how and what you do. You want to do well or discover why. But let the moment fade into time, and its humor will appear.

Your future milestones—graduation, career, family, death—are serious events sometimes happy and sometimes sad, but not what you consider today as humorous. Will you look for the humor in your daughter's future wedding, or wait for the photos to come back?

Relax with the moment. See it (and the future) from its lighter side, now. Find humor in the midst of an argument or golf game. Laugh at yourself. When things are heavy, smile knowing that at sometime even this event will have some humor.

Spread the humor of life on all that you encounter. You'll be happier and age healthier.

ARKANSAS

Kathleen Terrell
Age 54
Little Rock, AR

Dear Young People:

Can you imagine that having just three *bones* will help improve your life and the lives of those around you? All you need is a back bone, a wish bone, and a funny bone.

You must have a *back bone* in order that you stand firm for the moral absolutes that remain unchanged from generation to generation.

You must have a *wish bone*, that you will aspire to heights and goals untried by so many. Knowing that wishing alone doesn't make it so, you will be self-disciplined and work hard to help fulfill your dreams.

And you must have a *funny bone* to enable you to laugh at yourself and with others. It will remind you to give away smiles to friend and foe alike. Something as simple as a smile, your priceless smile, can help lift heavy burdens from the shoulders of those you encounter. You will be richer for having given away your smiles and those who receive them will also be enriched.

Bone up on life! What a wonderful world!

CALIFORNIA

Daphne Muse
Age 52
Oakland, CA

Dear Future Generations:

From my 108-year-old aunt, who was an ebony jewel set in the gold of modern maturity, and scores of others who never look back on their youth longingly, I learned to wear the patina of aging well. With the lines can come dignity, character, and comedy. Those mid-section gravity shifts may challenge earlier theories you learned about spatial relations. Multiple demands placed on your memory may require a regular release of irrelevant information from the "hard disk." Those silky, sometimes wiry, gray strands that weave their way into your crown are often indicative of evolving wisdom, earned honors, and prized privileges.

Healthy Aging is not a sentence to social or familial ostracism, fading memories, Medicare nightmares, or mere fodder for cruel, ageist jokes. Develop a treasure of friends with whom you build and sometimes rebuild relationships, and do invite those on the other side of the "generational river" to share in your life; often, they know a little about navigating upstream. You just may become the personal museums, libraries, and stories for future generations. Archive those memories well, preserve those precious artifacts, and share your stories.

COLORADO

Carolyn McNeel
Age 55
Golden, CO

Whether looking for physical, mental, financial, or social gain, there is one underlying foundation that all else must be built upon and that foundation is spiritual. I have learned that joy and peace must spring from a well within and cannot solely depend upon the circumstances, environment, or persons without. How we perceive what is on the outside depends on what we spiritually have on the inside. As a hospice nurse I took care of an elderly mountain hermit. His physical needs were many. His environment was filled with material possessions that were broken down, worn out, or used up. He wore ragged clothes, sat at an old kitchen table filled with dirty dishes, looked out of windows streaked with smoke and filth, and with utter contentment, said, "Isn't God wonderful! He has created such beauty in this world."

I was caught off guard as I saw myself, dressed in clean clothes, eating from a clean table and looking through clean windows, yet so often seeing only the ugly scars of war, crime, and selfishness of this world. The mountain hermit knew peace and beauty because he looked through the eyes of a spiritually contented soul.

CONNECTICUT

Phil LaBorie
Age 56
Weston, CT

Dear Chessie:

When I was young, my parents had a picture of a garden hung over their bed. In the middle was a saying — "Do you love life? Then do not waste time, for that is what life is made of."

I dusted that picture every Saturday morning, and memorized the saying. I thought it meant if I didn't want to waste time, I should keep busy doing things that are needed to be done. So I cleaned the garage, weeded the lawn, and washed our car every Sunday. I was always busy, so I wouldn't waste time.

Now that I am older, I think that keeping busy all the time is a real waste of time.

Some days we have things to do, but it's also nice to just let time go by.

That's why I sit and watch you finish your drawing before we go to the store. Or go outside at night and look at the wishing star. Or try to imagine what the puppy sees when she looks across the field.

I hope when you get older, you will want to waste time like me. You'll learn neat stuff if you take the time.

Love, Dad

DELAWARE

Joyce Reardon
Age 59
Dover, DE

I am 59 years old and am a very happy person. Life has not been easy much of the time. I have people look at me and think I have been very pampered—far from it! The single most important thing I would say to any young person is to never fear growing older. Look forward to it, the rewards are great and you do have lots of fun along the way.

As a teenager, I chose not to use tobacco or alcohol, to eat wisely, and to exercise regularly, and I had a deep faith in God. All of this combined got me through every circumstance in life. I am the mother of four now-grown children, and was a single parent and their sole support for a number of years. Just ten years ago I lost my home, car, business, and a large part of all I had worked for, but I had my health, faith, and dreams—all I needed to start all over, and I did.

I look forward to being 60, 70, 80, and yes 90!

DISTRICT OF COLUMBIA

John M. Howard
Age 52
Washington, DC

To Future Generations:

Gaining realistic information is the key to living a healthier lifestyle at any age, but as most of the problems caused by the lack of such information manifest themselves after 50, it is essential for the elderly.

A wise man once said that doing good is easy. The hard part is knowing what is good.

Why is it so hard to know what is good? The answer is that there is so much money to be made through the proliferation of untrue beliefs and ridiculous products that the truly good is forced off the screen.

The first lesson that we get is that the person with the most money or material goods or who looks the best, leads a more worthwhile life. When we simplify our lives as much as possible, instead of buying into all of the hype based upon this nonsense, we will be more stress-free. When we concentrate on food values instead of trying to force ourselves to be slim, our weight loss will be natural.

It is only by obtaining and heeding the true and disregarding the false that we can lead a healthy lifestyle as we age.

FLORIDA

Teresa C. Rose
Age 50
Mt. Dora, FL

Dear Future Generations:

As I reviewed the US Postal Service's letter-writing contest material and pondered the "single most important thing I wanted to share" with you, my eyes fell upon three little words, written in red, on the contest form: Write a letter.

Well, that was it! The answer to "what I wished to share with future generations" is: Write Letters!

Write letters to yourself to solidify your dreams.

Write letters to your friends to share their joys and sorrows.

Write letters to your parents to express gratitude and caring.

Write letters to your spouse to reaffirm your love.

Write letters to your children to teach, to bless, and to surprise them.

Write letters to your adversaries to forgive and to forget.

Write letters to Santa to keep joy and fantasy alive.

Write letters to the Lord that He may know the sincerity of your faith.

And someday, when future generations find your letters in their great-grandparents' attics, they too will share in the many life-lessons you planted on bits of paper through the years.

GEORGIA

Judy Hammett
Age 53
Stone Mountain, GA

I refuse to age. By giving myself to others I forget about the little aches and pains. I am a foster mom to medically fragile infants. With medical appointments, therapy, apnea monitors, oxygen tanks, feeding tubes, bottles, diapers, etc., I don't have time to "grow old."

I eat properly, lost eighty pounds, and take care of myself so I can help these precious little ones grow healthy and happy. When one finds a real reason to maintain good healthy habits, it makes everything in life fall into proper perspective. When we choose life over dying then we must also choose all that goes with our choice. Rushing from one thing to another, never taking the time to stop and "smell the roses," one day there are no roses! Roses must be planted, nourished, and loved. So must our lives be nourished. When we give ourselves to others, we find the "roses" in full bloom. Do not let death come in disguised as "age." Rather let life come disguised as the poor, lonely, motherless, AIDS patients with no one to care and the unlovable.

So don't go gently into the night but rather go out fighting.

HAWAII

John P. Moran
Age 59
Hilo, HI

A funny thing happened on my way to retirement—I remarried and started a new family. Certainly unexpected, a change in plans, something different! Without acceptance of change and enjoyment in the challenge of things different, "Healthy Aging" would be more difficult. Acceptance of change may be the single most important thing for Healthy Aging.

Certainly a good diet, moderate exercise, a strong belief system, forgiveness for wrongs done to you, thankfulness for the joy of each day (consider the alternative), dreams for your future, and maintaining an interest in people are all important issues for one to age healthfully. Each is a part of the whole of Healthy Aging. Some luck in the gene pool does not hurt either.

But, it is the acceptance of changes in your life that is absolutely essential for growing older healthfully. It is almost a certainty that one's health, relationships, institutions, or financial circumstances will change. Loved ones will die. People will move away. Favorite things may no longer exist. How a person accepts change is the single most important to their Healthy Aging.

Things will change.

IDAHO

Debby Deteving
Age 56
Boise, ID

Dear Daughters:

My brothers titled me "The Iron Woman" when Dad went to prison. My mother said I was just born stubborn because on my first day of kindergarten, a bossy first-grader told me the way home, so of course I went the other way and got lost.

I had help being stubborn. My parents never said "girls don't..." so I was the only girl in my senior math class. Marriage didn't stop my education because my mother-in-law set an example: Our husbands and children watched us march for our diplomas together. Dad and I acquired sons because two "disturbed" teens needed stubborn loving.

All of you stood by me when Dad went to prison. Those who said I should divorce him didn't know how we had worked, prayed, cuddled, and laughed together. Dad made the necessary changes in his thinking and behavior, and we began healing together.

Stubbornness, unless you go the wrong way—like me on the way home from kindergarten—substitutes for physical strength. In the worst of times, stubbornness is the iron rod that supports life. In the best of times, stubbornness creates enduring love.

Love,
Mom

ILLINOIS

Lois Sorkin
Age 56
Skokie, IL

The rivalry among the generations for preeminence on this planet makes Healthy Aging a lonely struggle.

As children we experience the world for the first time, and as parents we guide our children. By the time we make our third journey of discovery with our children's children, we understand life in ways that youth cannot know. Yet before we are ready to turn the planet over to these newcomers, they rush past us and stake their claim.

In fact, they are doing exactly what we did just a generation ago.

What we need is a reasoned perspective on our position—and theirs—in the droll, circuitous history of the world. Our reign ends and theirs begins, and both are too brief.

But what if we could share our turn graciously? Young people have fervor, dreams, and a fascination with the rush of events; old people understand the events because they have lived them before. What an alliance we could forge: One humanity, governed in tandem by the wisdom of age and the hunger of youth.

Early on, we should teach our children to honor, not denigrate, age. The whole human environment would be healthier—for all ages, for all times.

INDIANA

Janice Peterson
Age 57
Bloomington, IN

"If you don't use your head, you may as well have feet on both ends." This favorite quote of my father has encouraged me to "think" through many a questionable situation.

"Janice, always make five new friends a year and make certain most of them are younger than you," said my 99-year-old mother-in-law. It's quite a challenge to follow her suggestion, however, the proof of value was witnessed as the grandchildren of her departed friends shared Sunday breakfast at the table of Mom Peterson.

My own mother frequently reminded me with this comment, "Straighten-up!" As a youngster I felt it meant I should quit misbehaving, but as I mentally hear her voice now, it serves as a healthy recommendation to sit, stand, and walk erect with shoulders back. Thanks Mother—I needed that.

The joy I've received from this threesome is: Think for yourself and keep those brain cells active, share time with friends because sharing is caring, and always strive to maintain a healthy body by practicing proper posture.

I believe in their examples as I share them with you.

IOWA

Virginia Mortenson
Age 57
Des Moines, IA

As a 57-year-old woman; daughter of healthy parents in their eighties; widow of a teacher; mother; grandmother; teacher; school counselor; reader and writer, I have learned one most important lesson for Healthy Aging: *We have choices*!

At the age of 15, my husband chose "just one" cigarette—then, another and another, until smoking became a habit. Three years ago at the age of 54, he died of lung cancer. If only he hadn't chosen to smoke that one cigarette 40 years ago.

Now, every day I must choose whether to be miserable in missing him or go forward, making decisions that promote Healthy Aging for myself: Snacking on carrots instead of French fries; meeting real people or reading instead of watching TV; walking to the mail box instead of driving; realizing I'm in control of my thoughts as well as my behavior instead of choosing to seethe over social slight; reaching out to help others in the present instead of dwelling on past mistakes; laughing at myself instead of complaining.

Life whizzes by. Don't let yourself be whisked away early. My husband no longer has choices. I do—and so do you! Let's *choose* a life styled for Healthy Aging.

KANSAS

John Stuahan
Age 50
Topeka, KS

The key to Healthy Aging is learning to be aware that you are alive. After this education the next step is to again understand that you can maximize your health.

The alternative must be personal responsibility for a life less meaningful than possible. The more you remember the changes you did not make at 20, 30, and 40, failed opportunities. Reflection teaches one that changes made now could still make life better at 60, 70, and 80.

A lesson, watching the infirm old in a locked room at a rest home. A lesson, watching TV surrounded by a semi-circle of old women strapped in wheel chairs. They were being starved to death.

Do you want to be a zombie? If so, do nothing. Want to be able to *not* get into that chain, live now. There is still time, brother.

KENTUCKY

Jack Duncan Frost
Age 50
Bowling Green, KY

Healthy Aging.

The words just don't seem to sound correct right next to each other in most people's minds. It is time to change the way Americans think about the aging process. We have to begin to realize just because a body has been existing for more than 50 years, the warranty has *not* expired!

Regular *daily aerobic exercise* is the fundamental key to keeping your personal warranty in full effect. Just like any motor vehicle, regardless of price, preventive maintenance will always be the most effective *and least expensive* means of avoiding biological and emotional breakdowns. Aggressive walking provides an excellent means of accomplishing this goal. By walking early in the morning every day, I set the pace for my body's metabolism for the rest of the day, thereby ensuring maximum energy utilization no matter how demanding the activities.

Transplants, genetic engineering, and pharmaceutical breakthroughs may prove to add years to the average life expectancy—but it is a personal commitment to vigorous daily activity which will truly add *enjoyment* to a person's total life experience. No investment you ever make will surpass the dividends you'll receive from daily exercise.

LOUISIANA

Julia C. Mayet
Age 53
Cut Off, LA

My Fellow Young Americans:

It's all in the right *attitude*. Pain and suffering are inevitable. Misery is our choice. With the proper attitude one's health and well-being can be controlled. Faced with breast cancer in 1987, I was frightened of the uncertainty but determined that with the right *attitude* and faith I could survive. I did not let myself dwell on self-pity or even concern myself with the pain or the discomfort of chemotherapy. In my doctor's care, I fought back with all my strength, in physical therapy, right diet, prayers, and TLC from my husband and family.

I lost a friend to cancer. She was constantly negative and although I tried to reassure her that she needed to take control and change her *attitude*, she wasted precious time worrying about her survival.

My daughter says I don't act my age but, age is irrelevant, we are not limited. With the right *attitude*, proper diet, exercise, determination, and faith in God, we can do anything we feel up to, no matter what age we happen to be. It also helps when you have a loving husband who tells you each morning that you are loved and beautiful!

MAINE

Hannah Fox Trowbridge
Age 55
Brunswick, ME

Laughter is said to be the best medicine, thus a healthy sense of humor is one thing that I frequently apply to my own and others' aging process. For instance, people spend a lot of money tucking in their wrinkles just as fast as they start to hang loose. They miss out on the hysterical sight of their arm wrinkles literally flapping in the breeze on the window sill of their car going 50 MPH. I'd rather spend my time laughing at the inevitable instead of wasting energy futilely trying to prevent it!

With that energy saved, the next thing is to not self-limit activity due only to age. Keeping connection with family, friends, and new ventures continues along with full-time work. Rowing an ocean shell was unknown to me a few years ago. Now I find great delight in the recreation and local rowing races. I'm usually the only woman entered over 50 and win first prize in my age group! Wonderful fun!

Poetry-writing workshops, professional training, and many other diverse opportunities help my development in areas that I like but previously haven't had time to do. Balancing this rich aging process with growth and humor is continual throughout life!

MARYLAND

Armando Sandoyal
Age 59
Rockville, MD

Dear Guys (this is a guy thing):

Dance. If you don't know how, *learn*! When I was a kid I learned to dance because it was a great way to meet girls, now at 59, I appreciate more fully the benefits of dancing (girls have known this all along). Dancing is a plus physically, socially, and mentally. Simply put, it enriches your life because it is fun.

Where? The swing dances at the Glen Echo Ball Room in the Maryland suburbs of Washington, D.C. are very popular—the age range is from college to seniors and they have lessons for beginners.

Believe me, dancing is not rocket science. Yes, it is much easier to learn when you're young, hey if gals can do it—*dance*!

MASSACHUSETTS

Ruth Ann Rego
Age 53
New Bedford, MA

No More Worry.

From my wonderful family of fretting fanatics I learned to agonize over absolutely everything. Circumstances great or small, each was worthy of equal opportunity concern and dutifully worried over.

Well, that's fine and dandy when you're young and time seems endless, but this 53-year-old body is already setting limits. Worry is stressful and unproductive; it saps your strength. I can't afford to waste, with worry, any allotted time that can otherwise be filled with joy.

Try my guaranteed remedy for worry. Ask yourself, "If I do or don't do this, what's the worst possible thing that can happen?" If you can deal with the consequences, don't worry. Example: You're in your car, realize you're lost and will be 20 minutes late for the meeting. Will anyone die? No? Merely impatient grumbling? That's acceptable—so just take those 20 minutes to concoct the most blatantly ridiculous excuse to offer along with your apology.

Always consider alternatives, make informed choices, and plan carefully. Carry a road map, a car phone, and of course, always wear clean underwear. Then, when circumstances are beyond your control, accept and make the best of them.

And if all else fails, try humor.

MICHIGAN

Patrick Beal
Age 57
Stevensville, MI

Life is competition! People who train the hardest win the most. Health problems that go with aging are part of normal competition. Prostate cancer surgery is the same as any other competition—you train for it! I trained six months for prostate surgery and won the contest!

How do you train for prostate surgery? The same as you train to win any competition.

Prepare intellectually. I read everything available about the sickness, the operation, and potential complications. Physical condition at time of surgery was the major variable for winning.

Prepare emotionally. My spouse and I discussed how our life-styles would change after the operation. We agree to define winning as regaining nonsexual physical ability *as it should be* the day before the operation.

Prepare physically. I went on a diet, began daily workouts and lost 40 pounds. The day before the operation I ran 10 kilometers in 55 minutes, establishing a criterion for measuring recovery after the operation.

Finally, compete with someone you can beat! Within six months after the operation, I beat my 55-minute time for 10 kilometers. Recovery was complete—I had beat my competition.

MINNESOTA

Mollie Person
Age 56
Marshall, MN

Dear Future Generations:

Life presents marvelous opportunities. Instead of advice, let's look at observations gleaned over 50-some years.

You are the only expert on you. Be yourself, but strive always to increase your effectiveness. Look. Listen. Learn. Make a positive difference every day.

Enrich the world around you. Plant a tree, write a poem, assist a child. Share your talents; help others explore theirs. Anticipate. Educate. Appreciate.

Treasure old friends while making new ones. If family is the flour in the cake, friends are the spices. Applaud diversity. Be distressed by injustice, hate, and war. Cherish. Challenge. Change.

Seek peace within yourself. Use humor to diffuse difficult situations. Experience brings wisdom. Be passionate about your job. Measure success by results and how people benefit. Build a solid financial foundation. Laugh. Labor. Live.

Love your family, your neighbor, your god. Find worthy leisure pursuits. Take pleasure in small things—hobbies, books, animals, music, gardens. Dream. Dare. Delight. Volunteer for a cause.

Age is a state of mind. Enjoy. Envision. Excel. Remember the natural end of life is death, so make your journey meaningful, worthwhile, and memorable.

MISSISSIPPI

Jocleta C. Cartledge
Age 58
Kilmichael, MS

Aging doesn't happen suddenly. It begins at birth. The simple most important thing that I have learned about Healthy Aging is simple—look for something good in each day because it is the only day you are guaranteed. Instead of dwelling on the stressful things in your life focus your energy on the good things. Get out of your bed each morning with the determination to be happy. The only force we can totally control is our attitude.

In later years as an aid to mental fitness use your acquired knowledge to teach something to someone else. You know something you can share with a friend, child or grandchild; when you share with another your life becomes richer.

Insofar as your physical ability permits, stay busy. Sew a dress or a doll for a granddaughter. Prepare a meal for a working mother. Savor the mornings—the mid days, and the evenings. From birth to death take each day you are given and "rejoice and be glad in it."

MISSOURI

Carol Wibbenmeyer
Age 51
Manchester, MO

Asking for help is as painful as it is rewarding. "I'm not here to fix you. You have the tools to fix yourself. I'm here to show you how." With those words from my therapist at the conclusion of my first session, I knew I could succeed.

After spending a lifetime taking care of people, I certainly didn't need anyone telling me what to do; however, the roller coaster was spinning out of control, and nothing I did slowed it down. I knew I needed help for my survival and that I could not do this alone. If I had a toothache, I would see a dentist; if I had a clogged drain, I would call a plumber. Since I needed help with my "out of control" life, I called a psychologist. She listened objectively and never judged me; she offered tissues and a safe place to cry; she smiled when I began to realize I was worth the effort.

I am healthier now, able to distinguish between helping someone because of their need and helping someone because of my need to be needed. Christine, my therapist, was correct: I did have the tools!

MONTANA

Bettie Heeke
Age 55
Polson, MT

Dear friend, I'm writing to you on this day,
to ask if you will come out and play.

We'll play the game called "Let's Pretend,"
where we throw some caution against the wind.

We'll pretend we're kids once more
and go outside—right out that door!

Once we're out, we'll do something new
like hike, ski, or swim or just enjoy the view.

We're big kids now, and we're still learning.
Pretend it's our job to keep the world a-turning.

We can volunteer our help at the school.
Talk to the principal. He's no fool!

Teachers are stretched and budgets are slim.
Talking to youngsters gives back our vim.

If we don't go to school, we can go on a cruise.
Like Huck Finn and Tom, we've got nothing to lose.

The point of it all? Laugh out loud, have some fun.
Keep active and happy, 'cause "*We've only just begun!*"

NEBRASKA

Bonita English
Age 58
Red Cloud, NE

Dear Future Generations:

"Dear" in the above greeting is sincerely meant! At middle age now—through sons in their 20s and parents almost 90—I more clearly have perspective not only on the joyful exuberance and difficult struggles of your youthful years but also on the challenges that lie ahead. For this reason I share with you the following:

"Happiness is like a butterfly. The more we chase it, the more it seems to elude us." Accordingly, if throughout our lives, we continue to reach out in a giving way to others, it will become second nature to divine happiness from being "other-centered" rather than "self-centered." It is true that the way one is able to reach out generally changes, but what happiness even a whispered prayer, a little smile, or a kind word can generate through the generations!

The above key lesson on Healthy Aging, I believe, equals or surpasses in importance any physical or financial aspects, for the social dimension—the life-long pattern of reaching out to others—is the greatest boon in older age.

NEVADA

Stuart Pardee
Age 50
Gardnerville, NV

As a healthcare professional, I have counseled thousands of people. I learned early on to watch their carriage and look into their eyes. What I see often tells me far more than what I hear.

I have seen peace and joy in the hearts and minds of the aged whose bodies were racked with chronic pain, and I have seen pain and misery in the young whose bodies were healthy. What makes the difference?

The single most important thing is deep pride in who we are as a person and how we live our lives. This begins with integrity. Integrity: Uncompromising adherence to a code of strict moral values. Honesty, trustworthiness, loyalty, respect for the laws of the land, respect for others. Integrity transcends physical or mental abilities, and social or financial status. Integrity allows us to live our lives with a clear conscience. Integrity is our guiding light as we face the many and varying challenges of aging. Integrity frees us to love ourselves, to love our neighbor, and to love God.

In the truly healthy I see inner peace. It is ageless. Its source is love, and its foundation is integrity.

NEW HAMPSHIRE

Evelyn Amidon
Age 51
Merrimack, NH

To Friends as Yet Unmet:

I'm celebrating my 51st birthday today. It's not one of those big milestones with black balloons and Over-the-Hill cards. I'm past that and into the living of the second half of my life.

I walk the dogs for exercise, and put aside money every week for retirement. But the most important thing I do for my future happiness is to appreciate every day.

In a world of glass, metal, and concrete, I step off the pavement into the wet grass and soft mud, to catch the sparkling raindrop falling from the end of a birch catkin or rescue a caterpillar. I plant seeds and watch them grow, and savor the taste of a tomato still warm from the sun.

I hunt for dirt roads to explore, and stop and thank people whose gardens I admire. I have snowball fights and take walks in the rain. I hug the people I love and send silly cards for no good reason. I sing with the car windows open.

My body is growing older and rounder, my smile lines deeper, and my chins more numerous. And I am embracing the change and giving thanks.

NEW JERSEY

Mary-beth Boughton
Age 53
Summit, NJ

Having reached that ripe old age—fifty three
I'm full of advice—so listen to me
Staying healthy today is a full-time job
So eat your veggies and avoid the mob
When you're given a choice—as often you are
Go for a hike—don't sit in a bar
Drink plenty of water—it makes your skin glow
And wear your seatbelt—even when you go slow
See your doctor at least once a year
Call your spouse nice names like honey or dear
Spare yourself wrinkles—or worse—stay out of the sun
Resembling a prune is certainly no fun
Live each day to the fullest—and smile a lot
Mind over matter keeps you from going to pot
Don't allow your money to go up in smoke
Quit the habit before you're sick or you're broke
Have faith in something far bigger than you
When you climb the mountain enjoy the view
Love unconditionally and you'll always be glad
Acknowledge your feelings—both happy and sad
But the best advice after all the above
Is to keep doing something you really love
For very good measure always hedge your bets
Serve chocolate chip cookies with broccoli florets

NEW MEXICO

Donna Springsteen
Age 54
Hillsboro, NM

My Dear Child:

As the world begins to look toward a new century, I think about what advice I can give you to help you master this wonderful new future—where everything is possible, and yet, many things will be difficult.

All your life you will be told… "Be Careful…Pay Attention…Watch Out…Be Good…Stay Well" … all those two-word admonitions that are so well meant, but so tried and trite.

Nonetheless, I would like to add just one word of advice that will carry you in good stead throughout all your years.

My child, that one word of advice is *smile*. Look the world straight in the eye and smile. Smile when you say hello and smile when you say good-bye. Smile when you're in a foreign country. Smile when you're a stranger in a situation.

A smile speaks all languages to all ages. A smile bridges all gaps.

As you grow older, on into your own mature years, your smile will go with you, easing all burdens and brightening the lives of others.

Should you live to be 100, no matter what you must leave along the way, your smile will happily keep you company.

NEW YORK

Joanne Sherman
Age 50
Shelter Island, NY

Dear Friend:

You don't know me and I suppose you're not in the habit of accepting advice from strangers, but take a moment to read this. Because that's what it's all about—taking a moment.

When you're young and have a lifetime ahead of you, a moment may seem inconsequential, but it's not the years that round out your life, it's the moment; Like the moment you spend comforting a sad friend or listening to an excited child prattle on and on about finding a penny. The moment you spend actually reading an article about a healthy diet, jotting a quick note to that favorite relative you've just lost touch with, saying "I love you" to the people who need to hear it, praising a co-worker, calling your mother, watching a sunset, laughing so hard you cry—those are the moments that really matter.

Take it from someone who's older. When I look back it's not the years I remember, *it's those special moments*. So take your moments, use them, and invest them wisely. The return on that investment will be measured in something far greater than dollars. The return will be a happier, healthier, and more fulfilling life.

NORTH CAROLINA

Sally Ann Drucker
Age 50
Durham, NC

Dear 21st Century Americans:

For Healthy Aging, choose good role models.

For instance, my father learned to use a computer at age 78, demonstrating that it's never too late to learn something new.

Lane is another role model for me. Because her blood disease medication also created brittle bones, she lived in a body cast, taking medication through a chute in her chest. Yet she was consistently cheerful. When I asked for her secret, she replied, "I focus on what I can do, not what I can't."

Recently, I learned something new from my elementary school teacher, Mrs. Yearwood, now 91. Eleven class members surprised her with a reunion. As we celebrated in the restaurant, her pocketbook, left on a chair, was stolen. But she remained calm, saying, "I'm not letting one negative incident spoil a marvelous day." Class members turned 50 this year, but Mrs. Yearwood was still teaching us.

As I tell my own students, learning is a lifelong activity. Now that I've reached age 50, and aim for age 100, I look for opportunities to learn about Healthy Aging from the role models who are all around us.

NORTH DAKOTA

Jeanette Robb
Age 57
Ellendale, ND

Dear Americans:

The purpose of this letter is to convey to you why I feel staying mentally alert is essential for Healthy Aging. While your mental health is equally important with physical, social, or financial health, I feel the last three are greatly affected by the command one has of his mental faculties.

What can you do to maintain good mental health? Read a variety of materials on a regular basis; get involved in literary groups; keep on the "learning track" throughout your lifetime.

Read every day. Newspapers and magazines will keep you current with national and world trends, while stimulating the thinking and reasoning skills.

Novels can add pleasure to your life. Many new authors provide a variety of selections. Renewing acquaintances in the "classics" is time well spent. Joining a literary group will enhance this area.

Learning lasts a lifetime. Increase your knowledge of a favorite pastime by reading subject-related texts. Take a college course to investigate a new interest.

Keep your mind active. Exercise it with puzzles and games. Mental powers improve with age if you continue to use them.

In conclusion, let me reemphasize that maintaining good mental health can make a significant difference in your life.

OHIO

Clare Kathmann
Age 52
Cincinnati, OH

Dear Future Generations:

"I'm going to enjoy this decade," I decided two years ago, when I turned 50. I wasn't going to feel ashamed of getting older—as I had felt when I turned 40, even 30.

I've been lucky health-wise. And a combination of effective thyroid medication, a reduced-fat diet, and "power" walking several times a week has helped me stay slim.

But, nevertheless, life has brought challenges. After the recent suicide of a beloved family member, I decided to swallow my pride and get professional counseling to ease my emotional turmoil. This was something I couldn't tackle alone. The fact that we are social beings who need each other really hit home. It was a moment of truth—both humbling and beautiful.

I'm looking forward to continuing the journey into the years.

I believe that wisdom is a blessing that comes from learning the lessons life teaches. As we age, we may have a sore body at times, but we also have a soaring spirit.

Besides, our birthday candles give off more light each year. And we need to make the world a brighter place, don't we?

OKLAHOMA

Wes Bowman
Age 53
Ardmore, OK

Dear Future Generations:

Well, I hope you prepare yourself better for your future years than I did. Somehow I never realized that I was getting older along with everyone else. Those names in the obituaries weren't my friends' parents, but my friends themselves. That picture taken at the company picnic really did look like me. What had happened to all the time I had left? Was my financial statement correct? Was that all I had saved?

Suddenly I was 50. What if my pension plan failed? Could it happen? I couldn't start over. What if I couldn't work? All of a sudden I realized my future was shorter than my past and I hadn't prepared myself, or more importantly, my family for that future.

What to do. Panic? Give up? Never! Put everything off again? Tempting, but unrealistic. Make a plan? Interesting concept, but how? Try this.

Begin by talking to your family. Tell them your concerns. Get professional help on your finances. *Develop a plan*. More importantly, *follow your plan*. Even more importantly, *start today*, and while you're struggling along, think of all the pleasant experiences you had that got you in this mess.

Good Luck.

OREGON

Nancy L. Trotman
Age 51
Milwaukie, OR

Dear Friend:

Guess what I learned? To be needed *is* the secret to Healthy Aging—it really is!

About 20 months ago, my daughter, Holly, was confined to the hospital for nearly a year immediately after the birth of her second child—a boy. No one was available to care for the newborn except my mother, age 76, and my father, 80.

All year prior, Dad moped around—very depressed, his friends were passing away. All he talked about was dying, his will, styles of coffins, his burying place, etc.

The baby went home to Mom and Dad's house and he stayed a year! On weekends my relatives, friends, and I relieved my parents. Amazingly, my aging parents and the rest of us were all joined together by my daughter's tragic illness! Everyone had put aside their own worries.

My parents acted like newlyweds! "Their" baby brought them so much joy and *work*. We knew when "Dad's baby" got his first tooth. Dad had changed dramatically—he was young again! He was *needed*! As were we all!

Everybody's baby will be two this December, and *everybody* is very proud!

Gotta go—Mom needs me...

PENNSYLVANIA

Marlene Osheskie
Age 53
Apollo, PA

On my 50th birthday, I looked ahead and saw that, with longer lifespans today, I could realistically expect to see age 100, or another 50 years. I did not want to live those 50 years in this body.

Priorities were set. After 35 years of smoking, I made quitting smoking goal number one. My last cigarette was April, 1993. After one year, I added 15 pounds to my already obese body.

After studying nutrition, I began a style of eating that I knew would become a lifetime habit. I ate low-fat foods and walked for exercise. Within one month, I not only lost weight, but felt better than I had in 20 years.

Next, I got a job. I worked part-time at first; but now I have a full-time job with benefits.

As I head toward age 55, I am a *new me*!!

I quit smoking at 50.

I lost 75 pounds by 52.

I got a job at 53.

I have taken responsibility for *my life*, and I feel great. Come on 100!

The most important message is that "you are never too old to change your lifestyle to create a better style of life."

RHODE ISLAND

Shirley Fairbanks
Age 56
Providence, RI

To the Future Generations:

The best advice I could give you is to *think*.

Think—before you make financial decisions; listen to the opinions of others, and consider the consequences.

Think—before you make large purchases; don't be in a hurry to sign your name and make a commitment. Only you will be ultimately responsible for the payments.

Think—about the consequences before ingesting alcohol or drugs. This body is all yours for a long time. In addition, many lives are lost due to the impaired reasoning powers of drivers.

You won't always make the right decisions, but if you *think* before you act you will have a better chance for a healthy future both physically and financially.

In retrospect, looking back at my own decisions, some were made too hastily and later regretted. Sometimes I would like to turn on H.G. Wells' *Time Machine* and change some events in my life now that I know the outcome. Unfortunately it doesn't exist. But it's not too late for you. Seek advice, listen and *think* and you will be better equipped to deal with your life's decisions.

SOUTH CAROLINA

Lois A. Moody
Age 56
Garden City Beach, SC

The year I turned 50 I was diagnosed with breast cancer. I was lucky enough to have a wonderful upbeat oncologist who stressed the importance of a positive attitude. His manner was contagious and I found myself eagerly looking forward to the radiation therapy just to be around him and his staff. The disease took on a different tone and I became a survivor not only in spirit but physically too. My whole attitude changed and so did my life. I no longer played the part of the victim. I was now an active participant in my own journey. Life can contain some really rough roads. How you view them depends on you. Learning to walk these roads with a smile on your face doesn't take the rocks away. It just adds a cushion to the soles of your shoes and a bounce to your steps.

SOUTH DAKOTA

Alan Goodhue
Age 51
Fairburn, SD

Dear Young Friend:

I have had a wonderful life so far! Even my mistakes have helped. They've taught me that Healthy Aging is determined by just two things—Dumb Luck and My Own Priorities.

I don't always succeed, but here are the priorities I now try to live by:

First: Quiet Time and Prayer. Every day I thank God for my life! And I spend a few quiet minutes being honest with myself about my motives.

Second: Family and Health. Both are precious and irreplaceable. What I eat nurtures my health. What I say nurtures my family. What "eats" me harms both.

Third: Friends and Play. This comes before "Money and Work" because, the truth is, I'd rather play than work. And what kind of person would put money before friends?

Fourth: Money and Work. These are only important when I mess them up. The secret of work is finding a job I enjoy, whatever it pays. The secret of money is just to live on less than I make.

Fifth: Everything Else. If I take care of the others, I won't have to worry much about this one.

I hope this helps *you* set *your* priorities. And may you share my dumb luck!

TENNESSEE

Ariel Strong
Age 50
Summertown, TN

My advice? Acquire a sharp and well-made vegetable knife—the kind that with practice creates tasty meals.

And then, one day, with fresh vegetables and with that one excellent knife, you carefully and artfully prepare dinner. Then you invite neighbors and friends in for dinner and together you change the food you prepared with care and a sharp knife into shared memories and friendship.

Learning to use and care for a good vegetable-cutting knife teaches all you need to know about being healthy, about sharing, about staying away from sharp edges, and about love, the only thing you really need to know to have a wealthy life. Learning a useful skill with a fine tool and your miraculous hands will carry you through a lifetime of days and give you a way into the world. And then, someday, you will have something to teach another beginner on this journey of life.

So keep in touch and keep the peace. Be at home in the world and who knows? You may someday begin to tend a garden of vegetables with a finely crafted shovel to keep up with the demand for your skill with that one superb knife.

TEXAS

Diane L. Alvarado
Age 57
Fair Oaks Ranch, TX

Dear Future Generations of Americans:

A coping mechanism I use to avert emotional drain during stressful situations is an approach I call "objective circling" (O.C.). This procedure is accomplished by formulating a mental circle, placing a disagreeable person(s) and/or situation(s) inside the circle and stepping out in order to observe everything within it from an objective perspective.

Detaching oneself from the confines of the circle encourages thinking beyond our emotional being. It allows one to perceive the person/activity in the circle in an unbiased manner, devoid of personal feelings.

Words to avoid during O.C., if possible, are "you" (which sometimes rings to the time of "accusation") and "me" (a word often linked to "selfishness"). The third person tense works like a charm. An error on an invoice could be called to the clerk's attention as "there appears to be an inconsistency on this invoice," rather than "you made a mistake on my bill." This enables one to deal with the issue directly, separate from emotional involvement. Once emotion enters the circle, subjectivity clouds all reason.

Proclaiming victory over a battle utilizing negative emotional energy essentially declares us the loser. Engaging an O.C. attitude enhances quality of life, thus hails us as true winners.

UTAH

Judy Busk
Age 56
Richfield, UT

The most important thing I have learned about Healthy Aging is to decide how you want to age while you are still young enough to realize the pitfalls of aging. In my files is an envelope labeled "Letter to Myself to be Opened at age 65." I reveal the contents, written when I was 40, now, even though I am only 56.

Don't:

1. Become bitter because life wasn't all you wanted it to be—maybe it wasn't your fault.

2. Act like a bomb. Be your age—attractive, gracious, lovely, but your age.

3. Nag your husband. You've lived together all these years; why make the last miserable?

4. Talk about your operations, aches and pains.

5. Spend hours trying to figure out how to get one-fourth percent more on your savings. Spend your money on yourself or on someone you love.

6. Stop putting up the Christmas tree, even if no one comes home.

7. Spend hours looking through catalogues for bargains. You should be looking for better things.

8. Put up with unbearable things in your life and just "hang on" because you "have only a few years left." You may live to be 100.

VERMONT

Andrew Avery
Age 51
Jamaica, VT

Dear Future Generations:

It's possible! It's easy! You can do it! What is "it?" "It" is sustaining and improving your social and mental health as you grow older. How? By playing games!

In general: Cards, backgammon, chess, dominos, checkers, mah jong, etc. The thought process involved keeps the mind sharp as it plans strategies, follows rules, and adds scores. In addition, most of the games mentioned have their own groups that meet on a regular basis which gives great opportunities for making new friends.

In particular: Play Bridge! Bridge is still the most widely enjoyed game worldwide—according to the American Contract Bridge League there are currently nearly 4,000 Bridge clubs in North America with almost 170,000 members, plus an estimated 17,000,000 non-member players nationwide—and get this—the average member's age is 60!

Never played? No problem—there are books, videos, classes and even cruises available for every level of player. When you really get hooked, you can try to win masterpoints—an 88-year-old woman just became a life master!

Wow! Fun, games, friends, challenges! What are you waiting for? It's your deal!

VIRGINIA

Margaret A. New
Age 56
Middleburg, VA

Time has always been important to me, but when I turned 50, it became my most valuable, treasured resource. There will never be enough time in my day. On that final day I might well say, "Not today Lord. I haven't finished my list."

On my 50th birthday I treated myself, a single woman, to a spa weekend. It was a glorious, self-indulgent time of exercise, tennis, long walks, and yes, good food. I said to myself, at this juncture in life I can sit in my rocking chair and watch the world go by or I can participate in it. I came home to join a health club, embraced low-fat dietary habits, practiced tennis with a vengeance, and subsequently went on to two USTA national tennis championship play-offs. "I do what I love, I live my dreams, and I want others to work with enthusiasm." Through my business in career counseling, I help others find passion in their work and live their dreams. Life after 50 has been terrific: now I look forward to a challenge in my 60s...perhaps I'll walk the Appalachian Trail.

WASHINGTON

Alan W. Liere
Age 52
Spokane, WA

Dear Young Americans:

Healthy mental aging begins with the realization that age equals growth, growth equals change, and change demands a new appreciation. Though time has snuck up on me as it will with you, this is not a bad thing; I've not met a day I didn't like. To age contentedly, one must resist the temptation to compare apples and oranges and savor, instead, the uniqueness of each.

I had been conditioned to believe young was better—that I would sacrifice quality as I added years. I had been deceived. Young was the apple. It was good, but at 52 I tasted the orange, and it is good also. At 52, I do not have to agonize over my appearance, I do not have to look to others for approval, I do not have to prove I am a man. At 52, I can interact without having to judge and compete without having to win. I am not as pretty as I was at 18, but I am healthy, happy, and a whole lot smarter. When I was an apple, I had many questions. Today I have many of the answers. Indeed, the orange is delicious.

WEST VIRGINIA

Betty Joyce Champion
Age 57
Charles Town, WV

To me, Healthy Aging means expanding my mind to stay mentally fit. I was only 16 when I had the first of my seven children, so I never had the opportunity for a formal education. Now I attend courses at a local college, and at age 55, I earned an Associate in Arts, with high honors.

Keeping up with students less than half my age gives me a great deal of satisfaction. I enjoy staying in touch with today's young people, and I think my being in class helps to earn the respect of younger students for my generation, too. Of course, going to college means lots of home study as well as classroom work, so there's no chance of being bored.

When scheduling constraints keep me from attending full semester courses, I attend seminars, lectures, or short courses that interest me. There is so much fascinating stuff to learn and the more I learn, the more interesting and exciting life is.

I can't turn back the clock, but I'm making up for lost time and enjoying every minute.

WISCONSIN

Patricia Lorenz
Age 51
Oak Creek, WI

Dear Future Generations of America:

In 1989, I reluctantly invited a dozen women to my home so Sunny, who'd just moved to Wisconsin, could meet others who would befriend her. I was too busy to be her friend.

I invited everyone I knew...young women, older women, single, married, divorced. Women from work, from my church, neighbors, acquaintances, even the mothers of my children's friends. I filled my family room with lots of possibilities for Sunny.

That night something magical happened. Within minutes we were all chatting like old friends, laughing, sharing bits and pieces of our lives. Sunny exclaimed, "You women are downright interesting!" Someone piped up, "This is such fun we ought to meet every month and call ourselves the *Southeastern Wisconsin Interesting Ladies League*! S.W.I.L.L."

The Swill Gang has been meeting eight times a year ever since. None of our lives will ever be the same. Bold new friendships have developed. New women have joined. I learned the secret to successful aging...friendships with all kinds of people, all ages, races, religions, and marital situations. The Swill Gang keeps me young and feeling treasured by all our members. What a way to sail through the second half of my life!

WYOMING

Fay MacDonald
Age 52
Lyman, WY

Maturity and graceful aging is just the beginning to a wonderful, healthy, and active life. I attribute my healthy lifestyle to good diet, plenty of physical exercise, and a clean mental attitude.

The most important thing for me was becoming a vegetarian three years ago. Upon giving up animal products, I lost those unnecessary extra pounds, but gained so much more in energy and vitality. I enjoy waking up feeling great! I haven't had any illness, not even a cold or headache, for the past three years.

I now love to run. I didn't start until I was 50. Before I couldn't, I didn't have the stamina. I don't run fast, but I'm out there every day giving it my best and enjoying something I never dreamed possible.

Keeping healthy, physically and mentally, are the two most important gifts you can give to yourself. When you are physically healthy, you are automatically mentally healthy. You gain such a zest for life and a vitality for living that it surpasses all material riches. Being healthy and happy is the richest gift of all—life.

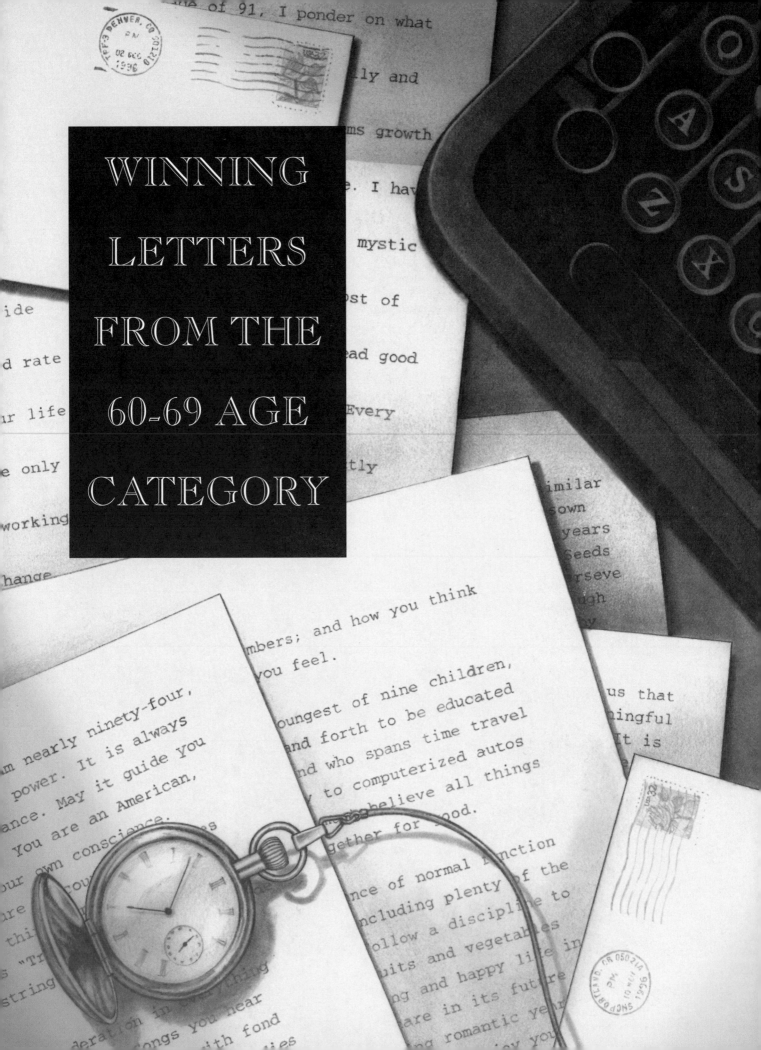

WINNING
LETTERS
FROM THE
60-69 AGE
CATEGORY

Robert N. Butler

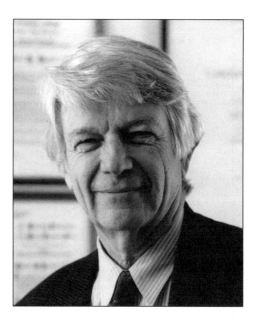

ROBERT N. BUTLER, M.D. is the Director of the International Longevity Center (ILC-U.S.) and Professor of Geriatrics at the Henry L. Schwartz Department of Geriatrics and Adult Development at the Mount Sinai Medical Center. From 1975 to 1982, he was the first and founding director of the National Institute on Aging of the National Institutes of Health. In 1982, he founded the first department of geriatrics in a U.S. medical school. In 1990, with Shigeo Morioka, he co-founded the International Longevity Center (ILC) (Japan-U.S.), which studies the impact of longevity upon society and its institutions. In 1976, Dr. Butler won the Pulitzer Prize for his book *Why Survive? Being Old in America*, which has been translated into Japanese and published in Japan in 1992. He is co-author (with Myrna I. Lewis) of the books *Aging and Mental Health* and *Love and Sex After 60*. He is presently working on a new book, *The Longevity Revolution*.

DETERMINATION

What an opportunity!—reading these inspirational letters from Americans regarding their thoughts about Healthy Aging. What an advantage it would be to younger Americans to have these forthright, interesting and imaginative perspectives. Among the many topics to which they gave attention were the understandable and conventional ones of appropriate financial preparation and good health habits such as not smoking. In addition they focused attention upon their children and grandchildren, family and friends, love and religion. But underlying and unifying all their views were a special sense of determination and of caring deeply about oneself, and by extension, others as well as conducting oneself constructively for the benefit of one's family and one's community. This may be quintessentially American, reminding us of the days of the Purtians, the dogged exploration of the West and the struggle of many up from slavery—each accomplished with a sense of community and the search after the "American dream," the very notion that one can better oneself and improve the lot of one's family.

These letters also enlarged my own perspective which has come to encompass four forms of fitness — financial, social, and personal, as well as medical. Most of us and most of our contestants were well aware of the need for good health behavior. Some were less aware perhaps of the importance of having a purpose in life, of productively, energetically contributing to society. Many did, of course. Many were also aware of the importance of having a social network, a body of friendships and relationships to sustain one in crises and in happiness.

What an experience, reading these fine letters!

ALABAMA

Billy G. Wesson
Age 61
Birmingham, AL

I would like to share this letter with future generations of Americans.

I am the oldest son of a sharecropper and learned at an early age about staying healthy, working hard, and eating balanced meals every day. Always, whatever job or profession you are doing, do your best even if the job doesn't seem important. Your rewards will be many.

Have a clean body and mind and when you meet that special someone, don't live together but get married and share this wonderful life with him or her. Nothing is more physically or mentally satisfying than living and loving with the same person for life.

We've been married since teenagers, she 16, I 20. For 41 years on our way to forever. Forty-one years, four children, ten grandchildren later, my wife still looks the same as she did at 16—I love her!

Socially, always treat friends as you would have them treat you.

Financial health will always be there with the above ingredients liberally sprinkled in.

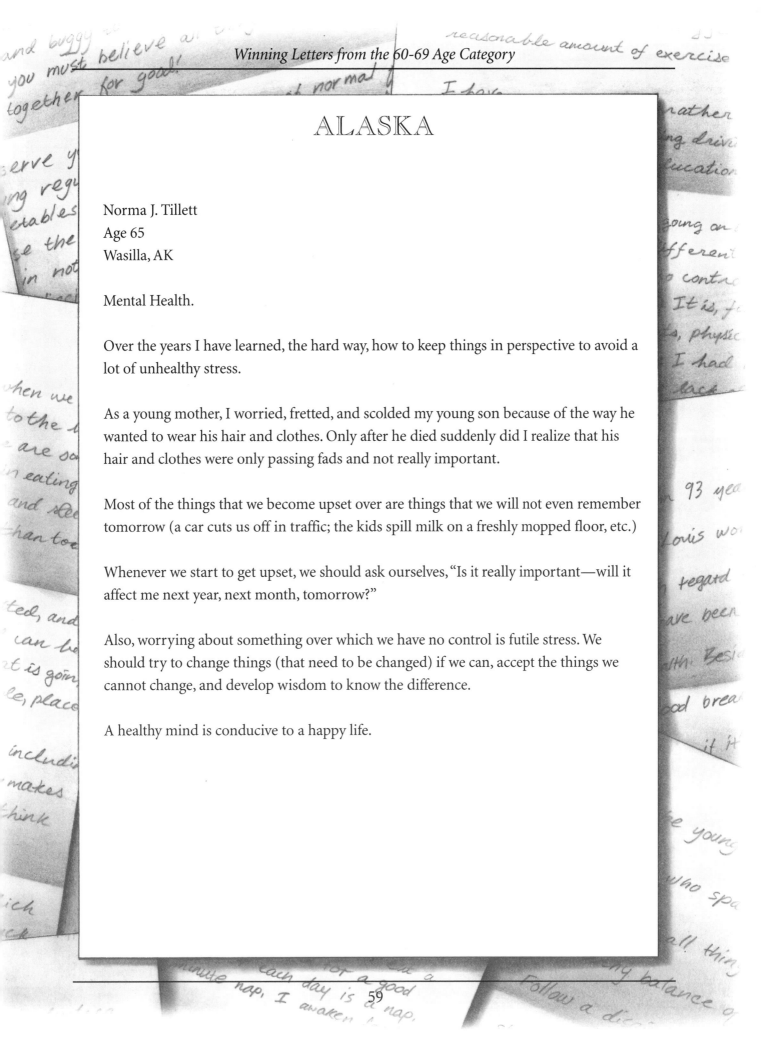

ALASKA

Norma J. Tillett
Age 65
Wasilla, AK

Mental Health.

Over the years I have learned, the hard way, how to keep things in perspective to avoid a lot of unhealthy stress.

As a young mother, I worried, fretted, and scolded my young son because of the way he wanted to wear his hair and clothes. Only after he died suddenly did I realize that his hair and clothes were only passing fads and not really important.

Most of the things that we become upset over are things that we will not even remember tomorrow (a car cuts us off in traffic; the kids spill milk on a freshly mopped floor, etc.)

Whenever we start to get upset, we should ask ourselves, "Is it really important—will it affect me next year, next month, tomorrow?"

Also, worrying about something over which we have no control is futile stress. We should try to change things (that need to be changed) if we can, accept the things we cannot change, and develop wisdom to know the difference.

A healthy mind is conducive to a happy life.

ARIZONA

Connie Spittler
Age 62
Tucson, AZ

Dear Special Ones:

Do not be afraid of growing old...for age is the great adventure...a trip that sweeps us along the currents of time. Take a deep breath and fly with the wind into each new day.

Reach out for the simple twist of mind and spirit that knows the answer: Participate. Now. This very moment. Jump into the fray that is life's daily offering. There is so much we can do...so many who need us. Things to learn...things to fix...sunsets to watch...soup to stir...seeds to plant...songs to sing.

This timeless magical way of living turns aging into a never-ending, always bending challenge. Adversity becomes a hill to climb...one step and then another. Be brave and begin. Participate. Appreciate.

At twilight...as oldsters...if we listen carefully, messages from the past reverberate within us. I believe the earth needs us to share our learning...to find our voices...give our wisdom...tell our stories. Opening up the one and only storybook we know by heart from beginning to end. Our own. Participate. Appreciate. And life will unfold the exquisite and curious wonders of aging.

ARKANSAS

William Laubner, Jr.
Age 63
Ashdown, AR

During my first 20 years of life, I learned from my parents and grandparents about love, work ethic, morals, and the importance of family. From my 20s through mid-40s, my role changed to that of a parent, implementing to my children the wisdom gleaned from my parents. From my mid-40s to the early 60s, I was labeled grandparent—interfacing with the new generations yet not interfacing in these subsequent family units. In my 60s, my focus became my parents, helping them to cope with their inevitable debilitating condition, and ultimately, assuming accountability for providing them with their eternal rest.

These 60-some-odd years have taught me that one of the major universalities of life focuses upon four stages of responsibility: Of a learning child to his parents, of a parent to his family, of a grandparent to his grandchildren, and then, to complete the circle, of a son to his elderly parents. Thus, life is a continuous evolution of responsibility. To accept cheerfully and with peace of mind life's ever-changing responsibilities is to accept aging with a healthy mind, a mind that encounters the traumatic shifts of role identification with ease and contentment.

CALIFORNIA

Jack Weinberg
Age 63
Los Angeles, CA

Dear Grandson:

When I was your age, I was taught that it was most important to learn the three Rs. Now that I'm older I've learned the value of the three Ps...perspective, proportion, and priorities.

It's not what you see, but how you look at things, for the latter determines the former. Aging will invariably diminish your vision but with perspective, will enhance your view. Your mind and heart should see more clearly as your eyes see less. Youth presents life in vivid colors, but aging teaches a new respect for sepia tone and endless shades of gray.

Before aging taught me proportion, I thought everything was important, but very little truly is important...or immediate. The simple, basic values of a life well lived, become increasingly treasured, and the pursuit of treasure increasingly foolish, for treasure cannot buy what you can bring to your own time with your own time.

Your children and grandchildren will teach you this if you haven't learned it before.

Once I understand time's limits and value, priorities shifted radically from wanting to change the world to avoiding the world changing me.

Finally, I'm wisely aging healthfully. Remember me.

COLORADO

Shirley Henri
Age 60
Ft. Lyon, CO

I had to learn to really listen to my heart—to trust my instincts.

I had girlfriends dying all around me at 50 years old because they were scared of old age. I said, I've got to find people who love being old and follow them around.

I found them out here in the middle of nowhere—two volunteers, one 93, one 90. At this Veteran's Medical Center, two of their life-long friends were honored for having more years volunteering than any other VA in the United States. I have amassed over 20,000 hours volunteer time here.

I discovered I need lots of friends more than I need lots of money. They taught me, "It's not how much you earn, it's how much you spend."

I still have my own teeth, sleep like a baby, and a 12-mile walk with my dogs on a Sunday afternoon is just a stroll. My goal is to play doubles in the Golden Master's Tennis Tournament at Wimbledon, England when I'm 85 years old.

There are still younger women dying around me because they have not learned one secret of Healthy Aging: "Volunteering!"

CONNECTICUT

Helen M. Younger
Age 66
Lyme, CT

Aging for me has been a most wonderful lesson in learning to live gently. Each year I become more flexible and tolerant, not only of others, but also of myself.

I no longer resent a difference of my opinions, but welcome another viewpoint to consider. I no longer expect situations to turn out exactly as I planned. More often than not I am pleasantly surprised as I've learned to "go with the flow."

I realize now that except for loved ones, every valuable thing in life cannot be held in one's hands. Health, time, love, faith, reputation, peace; these are the true riches of one's life.

So, dear generations to come, learn to live gently. Be tolerant of others, as they must be tolerant of you. Injustice cannot be cured by injustice, intolerance cured by intolerance. Be at peace with the world and live gently.

DELAWARE

Donald L. Kjelleren
Age 63
Wilmington, DE

"No Limitations" is a philosophy of life I've practiced for years. It is the best advice I can share with others. I believe no matter your age or condition, your dreams will come true once you accept that we have "No Limitations."

I observe far too many people who think and act like they are on the down-side of life once they reach 50, when the reality is they are entering their best years, the years of greatest achievement, well-being, and excitement.

Compelled to prove my beliefs, I embarked on my 60th birthday on a one-year high risk, never-before-attempted physically and mentally demanding adventure. After 76,000 miles of travel, I had successfully visited all 50 US states where I did a non-stop one-mile swim and a 10-mile run, bicycled 5,000 miles touching each state capitol steps, and reached the top of all but a few of the states' high points while raising about $50,000 for charity.

Having literally "walked the talk" I currently share the experience with groups of all ages. It is with satisfaction I can report that there are now many who now also believe that we have "No Limitations."

DISTRICT OF COLUMBIA

David Jickling
Age 69
Washington, DC

The most important thing to healthy aging is not to retire. Find new interests, new activities. There are so many ways that older people with more free time can help their communities as volunteers—organizing community activities, serving as guides at local museums, helping with church and club activities...

The rocking chair is the quickest way to senility and death. Each activity brings new friends, exposure to new ideas, and new challenges. That is what makes life worth living.

Too often the structure goes out of our lives when we leave regular employment. We don't have a regular pattern of getting up and going to work. We don't have a regular set of friends to see every day. Something basic goes out of our lives.

Being a volunteer—community helper—can make all the difference in Healthy Aging.

FLORIDA

Edmund F. Benson
Age 67
Miami, FL

This I have learned:

If you want to help yourself to success (which includes these three most important ingredients: health, happiness, and harmony), do things for others. Keep a Success Log and never let the sun go down without entering in it at least one thing you feel proud of. By doing this, you will develop what we call the "one success a day" lifestyle. Then, when things are not so bright, you can boost your energies by realizing you are a worthy person. Use these simple tools and nothing can stop you!

If you have invested in a good education and are willing to develop the winning attitude that comes from helping others, you will bloom wherever you are planted. But, please remember: No one can do this for you...it's up to you!

GEORGIA

Christine Burton
Age 69
Porterdale, GA

"Growing old is a bad habit which a busy person has no time to form." Andre Maurois said it and I am living proof that it is true. I was recently invited to join a club with a 46 age limit. My sponsor was shocked when I told her that I am 69.

The right parents help but keeping busy with important work is the most important ingredient for Healthy Aging. Sitting on one's duff and complaining about no one ever calling or coming to see you is the worst thing one can do. "Quityerbitching"—it makes you boring and could shorten your life—suddenly and unnaturally! Don't wait to be called or called on—get out and do something! Volunteer—go back to school—cruise the Internet! Don't just sit there—Do something!

Almost as important as keeping busy is learning to enjoy one's own company. If you live long enough you're going to spend a lot of time alone with yourself. How dreadful it will be if you don't like being alone.

HAWAII

Janet E. Powell
Age 60
Waianae, HI

Dear Future Generations of America:

The time machine is propelling across the world and leaving a cloud of dust behind, choking many who have known cleaner, quieter days. Internet is a shiny part of that machine, defining communication in a rush of instant answers, hurrying you to electronic cottages that house impersonal, mechanical teachers.

You must be strong. Strong enough to resist the pull of instant everything. Strong enough to maintain a steady course of involvement keeping you sensitive to your fellow man, resistant to the destruction of endangered species, and strong enough to be heard in the battle to save your children from products containing chemicals that interfere with their healthy growth and contribute to learning disabilities.

Get off that high-speed machine. It carries illness. Look to your spiritual health. Network with people who think of others and all areas of your life will improve.

When I became ill with a connective tissue disease, I thought my career was over. Disabled, I fought for balance and a new place in life. I began to teach others my skills and rest when tired. Balance brought a new kind of health that is stronger than my disease. I wish this for you.

IDAHO

Betty A. Anderson
Age 69
Idaho Falls, ID

A Zest for Life.

I have been involved in dance my entire life. The benefits that I have received have been tremendous. I have much more energy than many people my age that do not participate in any exercise programs.

Dance will increase your flexibility, along with improving your posture. Older people have a tendency to sink into the hips and knees. In a dance class you become more aware of pulling yourself up, and moving the body correctly; therefore becoming more flexible. *Life is movement*: and your thirst for living should encourage you to engage in an activity that will stimulate your body and your mind.

Take a tap dance class—it's fun, you use your body and mind, and mix with other people your age—this can be a tonic for the soul.

I have found older people often lose their enthusiasm for living, but don't let time ravage you. Have a zest for life and stay in touch with your body—physically and mentally.

ILLINOIS

Nilda Carlo
Age 64
Chicago, IL

My mid-life was sickly. I was working at a stressful job, tolerating a painful relationship with my then-husband, whining to pals who were themselves whiners and...stuck. As life and the mirror showed, my vow to age gracefully and in health—and to realize a lifelong dream to write—wasn't happening.

One morning on my daily highway commute, I drove beneath a seat belt reminder sign that blinked, "What's Holding You Back?" It startled me into naming obstacles to my dreams. I discovered I held beliefs about myself, life, and work that had forged attitudes which blocked me from living the life I wanted. I began to "adjust" my ingrained beliefs. Over time, I dropped the whining pals, ended the painful marriage, and retired from the job that devoured my energy. I took classes and began writing in earnest. I worked out of my home and had time for the children, grandchildren, new friends—and exercise.

I learned that—except for my beliefs—nothing holds me back. Now, I'm aging healthy. I don't accept "things as they are;" my senior years are an adventure; the mirror says, "it's only a number;" and...the only thing I don't have time for is whining.

INDIANA

Lota Henderson
Age 69
Noblesville, IN

Dear Fellow Americans:

Good physical health is dependent in large part on the absence of mental stress. After the death of my husband four years ago I decided to make a list of all the things that were worrying me and to take action to eliminate as much of that concern as possible. Not only did my actions free me to live a more carefree and healthy life, but it lessened the concerns of my children.

That list included the following items:

1. Make sure my will was up to date.

2. Place my handicapped daughter in a group home and make sure she would be well cared for. (Extremely hard to do.)

3. Bought a long-term health care policy to protect my assets.

4. Make a complete list of all important names, addresses, and phone numbers (insurance, property, investments, lawyers, etc.) and give to all children.

5. Sold my too-large home and bought a new smaller home. Much less care and maintenance.

What a difference these actions have made in my outlook on the rest of my life. I enjoy every carefree minute of living.

IOWA

Edith McAlpin
Age 67
Villisca, IA

The single most important thing I have learned about Healthy Aging is to take care of your bones! Women need to drink milk and/or take calcium all our life and get plenty of weight-bearing exercise such as walking or jogging.

Osteoporosis is a disease that can strike any woman. I did not fit the type of a small-boned blue-eyed blonde, which is generally considered to be at risk. I broke my hip in 1981 at the age of 52 and was told that I had good bones. In December of 1994, I shattered the top of the tibia and fibula in my right leg. At that time I was diagnosed with severe osteoporosis.

I am now under the care of J.C. Gallagher, M.D., a Bone Metabolism Doctor at Creighton University Omaha, Nebraska. He checks my bone density every six months. I am now gaining bone density by following his regimen of taking Tums, Vitamin D, Estrogen, and drinking milk. I walk for exercise daily.

I feel that every woman should have a bone density test by the age of 50 and younger if there is a family history of osteoporosis.

KANSAS

Lucile Hochstetler
Age 69
Hesston, KS

Risk Takers.

From Hesston, Kansas in the middle of the USA to Kikwit, Zaire in the heart of Africa is a big leap. My husband and I were in our 50s and had sold our business to become volunteers with Mennonite Economic Development. Our youngest of four children had finished college so a plan that we had dreamed of years before was set in motion.

The risk of leaving family, friends, medical, and financial security bewildered those we left behind.

After orientation we headed to France for language study. Our classmates were from all over the world. Some adopted us as grandparents while others included us in vacation plans to Southern France.

The culture shock on arrival in Zaire was a challenge. Life in Kikwit, the site of the recent Ebola outbreak, made us aware of the blessings of good health and the benefits of a healthy lifestyle.

We have been able to venture and dare to follow our dreams. We missed our grandchildren but the stories we have to tell them can't be found in any story book.

KENTUCKY

William T. Clark
Age 65
Vanceburg, KY

"Cross Word"—a "negative" for achievement.

"Cross Word Puzzle—now a "positive" image, something to challenge, perhaps to reward: drawing upon all our *past experience*, and creating a meaningful pattern. *Crosswords at our crossroads*—a metaphor for Healthy Aging, perhaps?

Recently I have returned enthusiastically to *Crosswords*—the large, imposing, difficult ones, which used to defeat me. Now I know or can *intuit*, most of the words I need—the happy consequences of a *Lifetime of Learning* (much of which was informed, unconscious, even subliminal).

We as *seniors* have a great treasure which the young have only partially: a *cumulative life experience*. This, when rationally channeled into pursuits that we find rewarding, can keep us interested in life and learning and interesting to others, even to young people.

Just as *happiness of the heart* comes from a life well lived and not from a determined quest for it, so *Healthy Aging* occurs as a dividend from a seniority well planned. Never stop thinking, reading, and learning!

Every minute is more precious now: Not to languish in depression and regret, but to flourish in the faith that we, not faultless but yet fulfilled, have served here some unseen greater purpose.

LOUISIANA

Nobie S. Makar
Age 67
Natchitoches, LA

Dear Future Generations of Americans:

The human body is a very special machine. We should care for it well. It needs good nourishing food, plenty of exercise (I walk four miles every morning), rest and relaxation, and most importantly, a very positive mental attitude.

I have no time in my schedule for worry. My policy for eliminating financial worry is to never buy anything unless I have the cash in hand to pay for the purchase.

I put love at the top of my priority list. It is what keeps me going. It is easy to love the lovable, but when we can love those who have undesirable behavior and those who are unfriendly, we are employing virtue. Sometimes it is very difficult to love our enemies, but we injure no one but ourselves when we harbor bitterness and hatred, so let us try instead to increase our tolerance, patience, and understanding.

I try to give something away everyday—a hug, a kind word, a warm smile.

I hope we will all remember to love our God, to love our neighbor, and to love ourselves.

I wish you a long, healthy, and happy life.

MAINE

Chet Gillingham
Age 66
West Newfield, ME

Dear Harry:

A few thoughts on aging as you approach retirement. I know your health is good and with your social security and retirement funds, you'll be OK but here are a few things that I think are important.

Learn to continue learning. Learn from young and old.

Share with others your experiences and talents when appropriate.

The secret of good mental health is to have no secrets. Talk it out with the family.

As the time draws near, remember, stay current with new technology, don't be left behind.

Laugh a lot. Make good humor a habit.

Seek out youth and stay in touch with them. They will give you years in exchange for experience.

Stay current with local, national, and world affairs.

Do enough work for money to stay active. Give money away if you don't need it.

Harry, this is important, learn how to quit. If you can't make something work out, and it doesn't really matter, quit. On the other hand, if it really matters a lot, never give up.

Remember to relax! The problems that you cannot solve, give over to another power. They will be in better hands then yours.

Be good to yourself. No one can care for you better than yourself.

Stay in touch. My best to the family.

MARYLAND

Mary Catherine Marshall
Age 65
Thurmont, MD

If I knew when I was young what I know now, somehow I would have changed my way of living.

I'd be more forgiving of imperfection in myself and others, if we had done our best.

I'd ignore an unmade bed and instead, write a letter to a friend or ease someone's pain.

I'd take more walks in the rain and make angels in the snow.

I'd know love is given, never taken and if not to be, set free for you can't chain a soul.

I'd not refrain from expressing love for fear of embarrassment or rejection for the grave has no voice.

I'd rejoice in friendship, but also, seek solitude, the salve that soothes the mind and soul.

I'd find satisfaction in success, but not worship it as the ultimate prize.

I'd realize yesterday is the teacher, today, the second chance, and tomorrow, a gift I may never receive.

I believe these things I'd do, if I knew then what I know now. Before the final curtain fell, I'd pray I played my part well and somehow, in some sense, I made a difference and someone, somewhere is better for it.

MASSACHUSETTS

Elaine I. McShane
Age 67
West Yarmouth, MA

There is a saying, "One must love himself before he can love another." I believe this bit of philosophy.

When my children were young it dawned on me that the best gift I could give them was to take good care of myself as well as them. This I knew because a sudden stroke had robbed me of my mother when I was a young teenager. Without fanfare, daily exercise, and good eating habits became a way of life.

Now that my family is grown, I realize that perhaps the *greatest* gift we can bestow on others is a good example. All three of my daughters are energetic women who regard exercise as vital to their good health.

It's a fact that taking reasonably good care of one's body benefits the mind as well. Still, none of us can ignore reports of violence or abuse occurring somewhere in the world each day. This is depressing and you need to remind yourself frequently that *most* people are law-abiding and kind to others.

So I would say to the younger generation, "Be your own best friend but look around always to see how you can encourage and help others."

MICHIGAN

Louise Bass
Age 67
Traverse City, MI

The secret of happy aging, like the mystery of the fountain of youth, is a prize widely sought after yet lost to many people.

For me, the secret was revealed when I was a child and it has given me youthfulness. It is an old saying that I learned from my mother.

Because I believed that adage, I am free—free of addictions and dependencies. Now, at the time of life when will power is weakened, I will not let any substance tempt me to excess.

I hike, ride a bike, paint, read, play golf with my grandson, maintain a home, serve my church, and communicate love to my family and friends.

What is the secret? It is summed up in a ten word motto—"Too much of any one thing is not good!" Sound simple?

It is the secret of enjoying the best life has to offer; sampling many things and not overdosing on any one thing.

MINNESOTA

Ken Lawrence
Age 66
Bloomington, MN

Don't let the world etch in granite the age of your retirement, for you alone must do the etching.

You hold the gun that signals the end of the game. The legendary soprano will not sing the finals until you push her from the wings to the center stage.

It is within your power to postpone the ultimate etching...To not fire the gun...To hold the singer in the wings. You can control all this!

True, your body may be slower, weaker, and less attractive now, but how fast, strong, and beautiful do you have to be to sing in a chorus, write a story, champion a cause, go back to school, or create a new concept?

Think of yourself as one of the "Un-group"...On the one hand you are the "Unfast," "Unstrong," and "Unbeautiful." On the other hand, you are the "Unselfish," "Unsedentary," and "Unstupid" and your life is definitely "Unfinished."

Instead of asking, "What will become of me now?" ask "What will I now become?" Set aside the concept of retirement and embrace the concept of graduation. The world needs you!.. Your productive life is indeed "*Unover!*"

MISSISSIPPI

D.W. Green
Age 66
Philadelphia, MS

When I turned 59 I weighed 245 pounds. I was diagnosed with high blood sugar, gout, arthritis, diverticulitis, obesity, high blood pressure, irregular heart, irritable bowel syndrome, high cholesterol, and arteriosclerosis.

In 1975, I broke my left wrist and suffered nerve damage. Surgery was not effective. I have feeling only in the tips of my fingers.

I was diagnosed with Parkinson's on January 19, 1993. I take 13 pills each day.

Today I am 66 years old and will turn 67 on October 20, 1996.

Today I weigh 155 pounds, I went from 45 in the waist to 34. My cardiologist says I am in great shape. All my numbers are average or below average. My neurologist says all of my vital signs are excellent and I am on the lowest amount of medication and have no signs of advanced Parkinson's.

I walk and exercise for two hours each morning.

My diet is low fat, low cholesterol, sugar free. I eat about two good meals each week. I make it a spiritual time praying for my church members and my family and myself.

Today, I have a quality of life better than I ever had when I was young.

MISSOURI

Dr. Ray Morrison
Age 63
Independence, MO

In many ways the human being is not so special. Many animals are bigger, stronger, can see and hear better, can run faster, jump higher, and live longer. What raises the human animal above the others is its unique brain.

The brain is made up of million upon millions of tiny cells. Those fragile bits of nerve tissue are interconnected and interdependent. There in that mass of tissue lies our humanness and our greatness.

Those individual cells must be carefully nurtured if they are to keep us above the beasts. They must receive nutrients that are necessary for their health—a benefit of a proper diet. They must not be weakened or destroyed—as a result of the use of drugs or chemicals often taken into our bodies fatuously. They must be bathed with proper amounts of oxygen—conferred by proper exercise and filtered through healthy lungs.

The heart may pump, loved ones may stand by, there may be fortunes in the bank, but without healthy brain cells, humans are a pile of dumb, useless flesh. Take care of those tiny little cells, my friend, for within them is your humanness, your greatness, and your joy.

MONTANA

Paul E. Hull
Age 61
Glendive, MT

Stand aside! You've been in the front line on the battlefield for most of your life, wondering when the breakthrough would come. It's here. Now stand aside and let those younger, fresher others have their time of glory. They are the reinforcements you always prayed for and you probably trained them. Let them have their day. You will still be a valuable warrior, but you don't have to collect any medals because you don't need them. Your whole life has been a medal of honor.

Stand aside and lighten up. This is the time for maintaining your own good physical and mental health, for enjoying all those wonders that you have taught others to appreciate, the time for laughing at the funny and the ridiculous, a time for boldly rejecting the unwanted, the time for being you again, not in a selfish but in a supportive, quiet manner that will enable you and others to get on with the rest of life.

Stand aside, please, and enjoy that great world to which you have contributed so much.

NEBRASKA

Betty Stevens
Age 66
Lincoln, NE

If you get two basics straight, then Healthy Aging is not only doable, but a pleasure.

1. Sometime, you are going to lose the battle. You will die.

2. Until that time you are responsible for your health—not your doctor, not how much your insurance covers, not some bad rap you got from your gene pool.

The assumption of responsibility becomes a most interesting way to live. It impacts your choices at the grocery and at the restaurant; how you budget your time to include some for exercise and adequate rest; what medical procedures and medications you will submit to. In other words, you're in charge, your health-care providers understand and respect that and it feels wonderful.

Good physical health is the best foundation for social, mental, and financial well-being.

If you lived forever, you would soon tire of everything. But knowing it will end revs you up to make it as good as possible until the game is called on account of darkness!

NEVADA

V.R. Scott
Age 67
Laughlin, NV

Greetings:

It appears to me that fitness is a very personal issue and matter of an open mind. A feller recently told me, "I've done this all my life and no young whipper-snapper is going to come along and tell me what to do!" It appears to me, that whipper-snapper may not necessarily be young and what we do may not necessarily be in our own best interest. Now this universe abounds with knowledge! The least bit of curiosity will get us onto that information highway—actually a luxury liner cruise on a huge ocean of miraculous discoveries—where we can compose a User's Manual to fit our very own body and life. We then become our very own whipper-snapper.

Then the best part is applying this "manual" to ourselves. As with the feller above, there'll be some "resistance to change" from those body parts—taste buds, muscles, nerves, even the brain—so, tell them to keep an open mind also. Before long, those body parts will be working together smoothly and we can once again do those things which give life meaning. It appears to me that's what fitness means.

NEW HAMPSHIRE

Randall F. Shaw
Age 65
Pembroke, NH

Healthy mental attitudes and practices we enjoy as we age are directly dependent on how we develop these mental attitudes and practices in our younger years.

We are motivated in our younger years to improve our minds by reading and learning new skills because of family and job responsibilities.

Exercising and improving our minds must continue as our job and family responsibilities are completed. We often have more time available. Our children are older and becoming self-sufficient and our jobs are often less demanding of our time and efforts.

This is when many new opportunities become available to us. I was able to enroll in adult education classes at a local community college. I completed courses in literature, history, statistics, computer language, and several other courses that challenged my mind. It also broadened my interest in new areas.

I became active in our government by serving in several volunteer positions. I also became more active in fraternal and veteran organizations and many of the community activities that they support.

Our physical, social, and financial health are directly dependent on our mental health. Please take advantage of all the opportunities that we have to improve and maintain our mental health.

NEW JERSEY

Catherine G. Lane
Age 65
Bayonne, NJ

Once a long time ago, my thoughts turned to the future. I was 23 and my husband was 24. It was the day we returned from our honeymoon 43 years ago.

After being carried over the threshold of our apartment and unpacked, we sat down and relaxed with a cup of tea and thought about our future.

My young husband asked what my wishes were. I knew our love for each other would get us through anything and it did; we were always healthy, we had good families and many friends—what could I wish for? My exact words were "...plan for our financial security for our senior years so as not to be a burden to our future children..." He did just that! We treated our savings as the bill to be paid first each month. His financial ability with stocks and bonds was amazing. We educated three children, built a new home, and he was able to retire at 56. Today at 66 I'm a widow, lonely, but financially secure and happily helping my children financially.

My advice is plan for your future when you are young and trust in God.

NEW MEXICO

Jewell Johnson
Age 63
Las Cruces, NM

As a child growing up I learned the secret of Healthy Aging from my mother. She fed every transient that knocked at our door. Loaves of her homemade bread were freely shared with our neighbors. Often the unfortunate and forgotten people of the town dined at our table.

By her example I found that I will be healthier and happier when everyday I give myself away in helping others.

I've followed in her steps by working in a shelter for abused women and teaching children in my church.

Opportunities to help others are unlimited. America's children need tutors in school. Churches, synagogues, boys' and girls' clubs, and kids' sports programs need a constant flow of workers.

We can help adults by volunteering in nursing homes, libraries, hospitals, soup kitchens, and homeless shelters.

The entertainer Danny Thomas said, "In this world there are 'givers' and 'takers.' The 'takers' eat better, but the 'givers' sleep better."

By forgetting the big "I," by not asking, "What's in it for me?" by being a "giver," we discover the secret of Healthy Aging—and of life.

NEW YORK

Walter Rosenbaum
Age 67
Cambridge, NY

The key to Healthy Aging, to successful living, is to reduce stress wherever you can control the situation.

The formula: Don't Do What You Don't Want to Do.

Don't go where you really don't want to be: Your presence will be a negative one.

Don't continue an unhappy relationship. It will make you both sick, and any children involved will suffer because of it.

Don't keep a job that you dread going to every day. Your future is not engraved in stone. You can change. There are options, but you have to seek them out, be it a change in career or lifestyle. An unhappy lawyer can become a successful fisherman, if that's what he wants. A discouraged farmer can transform into a knowledgeable stockbroker, if he's willing to put in the years of training required.

You can meet other people, or be alone if that is your dream.

There are few people who make it to old age carrying bad relationships and bad jobs on their backs. This is America! You are free to pursue your dreams. Get out of the rut leading to nowhere!

NORTH CAROLINA

Ernest Mazzatenta
Age 64
Hendersonville, NC

Reaching 65 doesn't have to mean that your brain cells atrophy. It's all up to you. I have found that what I learned and practiced before retirement is a solid foundation for what I am learning and doing now. Having written and edited throughout my business career, I had an urge to pass on what I knew, and in the process, add to it. So I sought out and eventually located a college teaching job that allows me to help a younger generation communicate more effectively.

Preparing for class—and listening to my adult students — have not only enlarged my understanding of communication but increased my appreciation of adult learners. Oftentimes after class, I feel greatly enriched by student insights, experiences, and opinions. What a delightful bonus! Had I simply retreated to a golf course, none of these golden-year "goodies" would have been mine.

To those reaching 65 (or anyone reaching retirement) I say this: Refuse to fall apart mentally—and you won't. If you build on what you know, if you seek out and really listen to those who are younger, you can remain as mentally agile, and as interesting to others, as you have ever been.

NORTH DAKOTA

Jean J.E. Walterson
Age 65
Jamestown, ND

Dear Jay:

You're just about to go from being a teenager to being what we can legally call an adult. Before you know it, you could become a husband, a parent, soon a grandparent and you'll think the prospects are that you might feel as old as you think I am right now.

Life is interesting. This old grandmother doesn't have any aches and pains that she didn't have 40 years ago. You won't either if you take care of your health now, and continue to do so as life moves along the escalator to the grayness of maturity.

You don't have to go out and play tackle football, or jog too many miles a day, or bench press your own weight to keep healthy. Barring accidents and serious disease, if your mind is young and active and you keep it smiling and working, the rest of you will never grow into old decrepity. Happiness is a choice that we can all make, and with happiness comes better health.

Respect the rights of others, and help them to respect yours. Be honest, play fair, and keep safe. Above all, help yourself and others to seek true happiness.

Your Grandmother

OHIO

Donna Scotten
Age 68
Columbus, OH

Every Day is a Holiday.

In 1971, the doctors told me I had cancer. I was terrified for myself and my family. I still had so much to do, three children in school so I didn't have time for this dreadful news. After many tears and prayers it was decided I should have 21 radiation treatments and a four day radium implant. Through all this I asked God to please give me the courage and strength to see this treatment to the end plus to please give me enough time to see my children and grandchildren grow up.

I vowed I would treat every day from then on as a gift, for it's a holiday.

I meet the morning with excitement and anticipation of a wonderful gift, "another day." I try to share my joy with others for mental outlook and attitude are the most important assets I have.

To enjoy life you must have a positive attitude and let your friends know you cherish every day and thank God for giving you additional time to love, care, and share.

Remember "Every Day is a Holiday."

OKLAHOMA

Dolores White
Age 64
Durant, OK

People are the same. Take away the language barrier and we're alike. Visiting the villagers in the Stavropol region of Russia, my line of communication was an 18-year-old interpreter.

I had studied about Russians. I read books on persecution from the communists. While speaking, I watched people nodding their heads. Tears streamed down the wrinkle-lined faces of older women. When I finished, a woman told me her husband had been sent to prison in '37, never to be heard from. Later, she handed me a picture of herself. A message written in old Russian covered the back.

Others told of imprisonment.

The people accepted me. They gave me gifts ranging from dried fish to a carved wooden box which contained drawings and written history of the village. I felt humbled when I read the sign, "Well come the guest from America," but the offer to build me a house, so I could live among them, proved to be the greatest gift.

I might say, "I'm too old to travel to Russia." Thankfully, I didn't. I experienced one of the greatest events of my life...so touching, three months later, I returned for another visit.

OREGON

Bob Holtel
Age 65
Ashland, OR

Shortly after my 53rd birthday, I began a multi-day trial run—to run the Pacific Crest Trail from Mexico to Canada.

No one had ever done this. It is a long way—2,638 miles—not counting side trips to resupply. This trek will ultimately impact my life more than any other conceivable activity. I would achieve a spiritual awareness I'd never even considered.

I became an uncertain intruder in unfamiliar territory. My arduous itinerary entailed running, on the average, a marathon a day for 110 days. One 15-pound fanny pack was my entire material word for five months. The life I left behind would never be viewed in exactly the same way.

The physical hazards would be many. Also, I had to cope with overwhelming emotional trauma and loneliness. The physical activity enhanced my mental state. I sought, fought, and survived the intensity of a monumental task. Our most innate rewards stem from persistent struggle.

This day to day effort and its cumulative effects have prioritized and purified my lifestyle. By comparison, any current problem seems insignificant. My senses are forever altered.

What is your personal challenge? Will it begin today, tomorrow, or never?

PENNSYLVANIA

Rose Marie Lorentz
Age 61
Lansdale, PA

It's challenging to write a lifetime of advice in 200 words.

The greatest joy in my life was having and raising two wonderful sons. The greatest achievement was learning to love myself. If you can love and respect yourself, you will have something no one can take away from you. It is more valuable than all the riches in the world. Loving yourself does not mean excluding others. Our family and friends are our support system just as we are theirs. By making someone happy, you will be happy too.

If you love yourself, you will take care of your body by not putting anything into it that you'll regret later—drugs, alcohol, nicotine, fatty foods. Now chocolate is the exception. It is the only obsession allowed. But necessary, especially in times of stress. There's nothing like a chocolate bar after a bad hair day or trying day at the office.

Look to a Higher Being, especially when life deals a blow that knocks you to the ground. You'll find there is someone up there, beside you, inside you. If you just slow down long enough, take a deep breath, relax, you'll find Him/Her.

RHODE ISLAND

Olga S. Toulmin
Age 63
Providence, RI

What a difficult question—the *single* most important thing I have learned about Healthy Aging. So many factors such as courage and optimism make a difference, but I would like to share with you why I think learning a new skill is most important.

Recently a friend and I presented a slide show documenting the history of a small town in Maine. We had little money but because my friend taught herself to use a copy stand to take pictures we were able to assemble over 300 slides of old snapshots and postcards that were loaned to us by some of the local residents. The show and script produced a record-breaking audience, a grant from the Maine Humanities Council and publicity beyond our wildest dreams. A young reporter was amazed that my friend had taught herself how to photograph memorabilia for slides. Perhaps a key lesson is that we should all exercise the talents we have as we age, but to learn to do something completely new requires imagination and a can-do attitude that is the basis for successful aging. Whoever said, "You can't teach an old dog new tricks?"

SOUTH CAROLINA

Lewis Tisher
Age 64
Charleston, SC

There is an ancient story about food, water, and air debating their importance. Air won, because it was the most important. Air's absence strikes first.

I would like to share a comparable lesson about aging. We age socially, mentally, and physically. If these areas of aging were to debate, there would be important facts for each.

Socially we interact. Mentally we respond. One, however, is most important. Without this one we could not have others. Physical health is like air.

Without air we could not act nor interact. We could think, but it would be idle speculation without movement.

Physical health, besides being the mover for the others, is easy to maintain. Exercise can be taken with no cost. Reward and improvement can be measured to the smallest degree and the feedback from such effort is rewarding.

The activity the body thrives on is use. Lack of use is automatically a sentence. Use is automatically a reward. Use is the factor that ensures. Without use nothing is possible.

Exercise to whatever extent is possible. Harvest the rewards and take pride in the accomplishment.

SOUTH DAKOTA

Alice Davidson
Age 62
Pierre, SD

Dear Friends:

It didn't occur to me I was getting older until a great gal suggested I write this letter on Healthy Aging. I'm busy living my life, not just existing in it. I hadn't bothered to think about time frames or stages my life fit into. She's right, however, I am aging and it's OK.

Young, when my mother was making funeral arrangements for her mother, I remember vividly her many remarks of things unsaid and undone between them. She was tormented by the knowledge this could not be resolved.

Not wanting that kind of torment, I was determined to live today doing the things needed to be said and done, thereby, automatically protecting tomorrow.

Unknowingly, that philosophy has been a factor and has fit all aspects and stages of my life. From interacting with friends to saving a dollar, from marriage and raising a family, and an outside job to retiring and aging.

I live, not just exist. I'm part of whatever I do.

This turned into a story rather than a letter. Must be the Irish in me. Good luck to us all on our journey for whatever days make up our lives.

TENNESSEE

Bettylene Franzus
Age 68
Johnson City, TN

The most important requirement for Healthy Aging is a emotion and mental attitude which says "My life is still worth living and learning."

Given adequate food and shelter, it is the emotional and mental approach which renders Healthy Aging a possibility. My approach has been to return to college to pursue a doctorate in education.

Education, regardless of whether it is for personal pleasure or enlargement of one's appreciation for areas of information not visited earlier in life, whether it is for a degree in a new field or an extension of earlier studies, is the key to staying mentally alert. It doesn't matter a whit whether the newly-found interest is in Asiatic Cookery, Ceramics, Quilting, getting a General Education Degree (if you haven't finished high school), or starting a college program. Using one's brain on a continual basis has been found to help older folk retain their ability to cope with advancing aging of the body.

My degree should be finished in the spring of 1998 when I will be 70 years old. After I get my degree I plan to try for the Peace Corps, Vista Volunteers, or some other service organization. Going my way?

TEXAS

Herbert Piller
Age 61
Georgetown, TX

Over the years, I have learned that I must accept things I cannot change. I must worry about things less. Getting fired can be the best thing. There's really no bargain at a cheap price. I must always say "Thank you" and "Please." I am only as good as my word. Money isn't everything. It doesn't cost anything to be nice. Nothing comes without effort. Children and grandparents are a great combination. You don't tell your pains to others. Love is the greatest treasure of all. You can't hug your loved ones too much. I can't expect others to solve my problems. If you care, it shows. A donkey dressed in a tuxedo is still a donkey. You don't look back, except to learn a lot. My mother and father are always happy to see me. Self-pity is a waste of time. Life sometimes gives you a second chance. A good reputation is my greatest asset. Everybody is attractive if they smile. Wealthy people are no happier than poor people. I should never pay for a job till it's completed. Days are long, but life is short. Good health is true wealth. Opponents should make up as quickly as possible.

UTAH

Joan Martin
Age 60
Orem, UT

This is me in a field of Kansas sunflowers in August at age 59 and today, the 24th of September, 1996, I am 60 years old! I would like to give inspiration to upcoming generations by encouraging them to be kind and generous to others as well as themselves. Kindness in our everyday dealings yields rewards: You can bank on it. You can't be too kind or generous.

Kindness to yourself is what you deserve first. This is the fuel in your tank that will drive your life. When you are kind and gentle on your self, you will be kind and gentle to others, whether it is children, peers, the little guy, or your hero. Kindness opens hearts and doors. You can have money, notoriety, and fame, but without kindness and generosity these assets will not sustain you as you age. You need only not to give kindness, but to receive it as well to survive. Kindness will show in your face physically, keep your mind healthy, and bring you good fortune. Today as I blow out those candles, I couldn't be happier. I thank you for your kindness for inviting me to share my thoughts.

VERMONT

Gretchen Besser
Age 67
Morrisville, VT

Dear Future Americans:

No gift is more blessed than good health. As long as possible, remain physically and mentally active. Eat and drink in moderation. At age 67, I weigh what I did at 20, having turned vegetarian two years ago. I stopped smoking when pregnant with my first son, now 42. Don't even start. For sport, I downhill ski (and kid myself I'm improving), horseback ride, do low-impact aerobics, and hike the Green Mountains.

The finest counterbalance to physical endeavors is intellectual exercise. Even crossword puzzles provide mental gymnastics. To continue teaching at college via computer conferencing, recently I had to learn about the Internet and the Web. I've written five books (the last one published when I was 65) and am working on a sixth. Striving toward a goal, however late in life, keeps you on your toes and staves off boredom.

Serenity is a beautiful if elusive goal. Age may not have endowed me with wisdom, but it has mellowed my outlook. I thank God daily for His blessings. Whatever your beliefs, some form of spirituality is essential to achieve equanimity.

Remember Juvenal's *mens sana in corpore sano*. Strike a golden balance, and your later years will be golden.

VIRGINIA

Geraldine B. Jones
Age 66
Chester, VA

After my retirement three years ago, I started out still trying to work all the time; I opened a home-based technical writing business and did consulting work; I ran constantly when I wasn't working, looking for something, afraid of staying home long enough to get bored.

After a year or so, I also started taking aerobics, learning bridge, walking, working at my hobby restoring dolls, taking computer and desktop publishing classes, and doing technical writing and graphic design work for church, family, and friends. After 26 months, I suddenly realized I was busy, happy, contributing to others, getting more exercise than ever before in my life, and feeling well and was content with myself and my life.

Being content with yourself, or knowing who you are and accepting it, is the best thing that can happen to you in your senior years; and it usually comes through age and experience. It's being comfortable with yourself and not worrying about other people's perceptions. It's being able to say, "I am what my whole life has been: Upbringing, genes, education, parenting, profession, and environment" and being able to be comfortable with that knowledge.

WASHINGTON

Sherman Kirkham
Age 69
Bellevue, WA

It's true. There is a secret to healthy, vigorous longevity. When you discover it, your life will become an exciting adventure. Tomorrow will be greeted with a spirit of great hope and anticipation.

The answer is simple: Reach out for that one thing you have always wanted to do, no matter how lofty or improbable. Then visualize success as though it were yours, beginning the journey with that first bold step. Fix this goal in your imagination and believe in it. Then anticipate, anticipate. It will change your tomorrow and every day thereafter.

Anticipation is the most magnificent emotion of all. It has built bridges, buildings; it has written songs and books and poetry. Anticipation will make you glow with energy and enthusiasm. Your vigor and determination will attract all those with whom you come in contract. They will want to be with you and help you. All good things will come your way.

You have never been more needed, more capable, more worthy. You are a national treasure. You will have found the greatest fountain of youth in existence. Use it. The world will be richer when you do.

WEST VIRGINIA

Nancy Hayes Hamm
Age 67
Point Pleasant, WV

I haven't found a fountain of youth but I have found a fountain of healthy attitudes. You're invited to drink from this fountain.

First drink of *commitment*. You must commit yourself to a healthy diet and regular exercise if you want to age healthily.

Next take a big drink of *friendliness*. Be amicable. Do something nice for someone else at least once a week. Go out. Get involved in activities that you enjoy. Don't wait for others to come to you. Go to them. If you make others happy, you will be happy too.

Drink of *contentment*. Learn to be content with what you are and what you have. Spend only what you can afford. Do not buy on credit except for a home or automobile. Start saving part of your income as early as possible to ensure financial health in later years.

Take a big drink of *faith*. Trust in God. Have faith that if you do your part God will do more than you ever dreamed.

This fountain never runs dry so drink again and again to keep a healthy attitude.

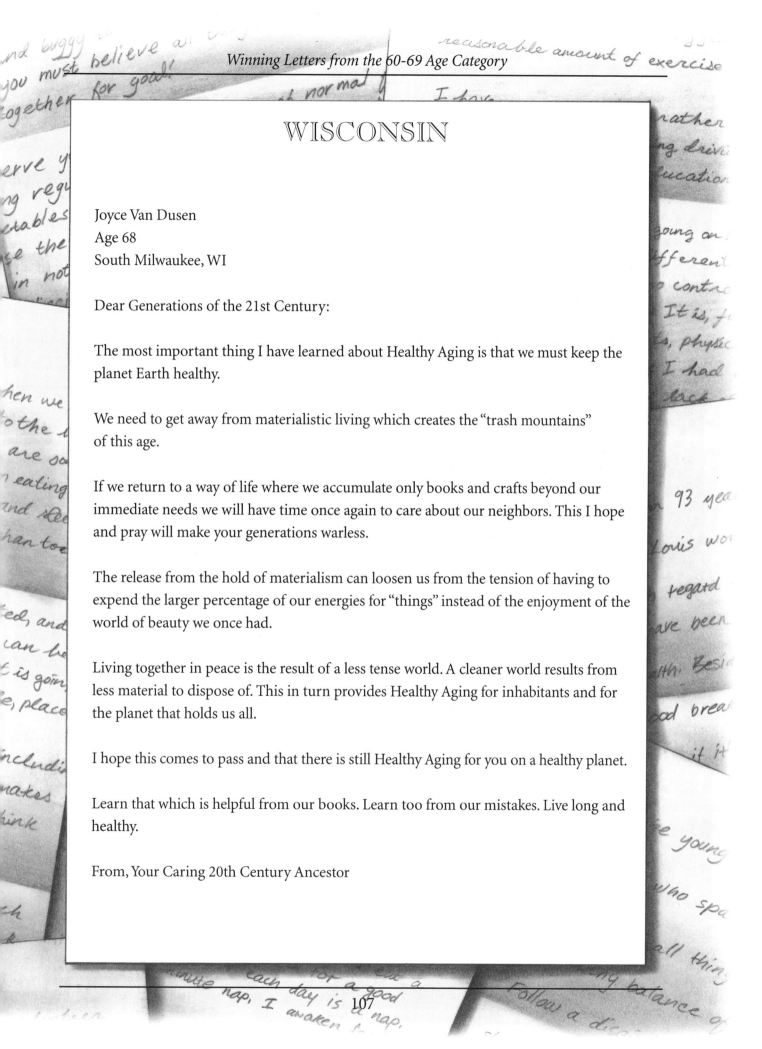

WISCONSIN

Joyce Van Dusen
Age 68
South Milwaukee, WI

Dear Generations of the 21st Century:

The most important thing I have learned about Healthy Aging is that we must keep the planet Earth healthy.

We need to get away from materialistic living which creates the "trash mountains" of this age.

If we return to a way of life where we accumulate only books and crafts beyond our immediate needs we will have time once again to care about our neighbors. This I hope and pray will make your generations warless.

The release from the hold of materialism can loosen us from the tension of having to expend the larger percentage of our energies for "things" instead of the enjoyment of the world of beauty we once had.

Living together in peace is the result of a less tense world. A cleaner world results from less material to dispose of. This in turn provides Healthy Aging for inhabitants and for the planet that holds us all.

I hope this comes to pass and that there is still Healthy Aging for you on a healthy planet.

Learn that which is helpful from our books. Learn too from our mistakes. Live long and healthy.

From, Your Caring 20th Century Ancestor

WYOMING

Donna Lee Sharp
Age 61 and 7 months
Lander, WY

Dear Future Friends:

The most important thing I can share with you about Healthy Aging is "practice who you want to be."

If you understand that you create who you are by what you give to others and to yourself, your aging process is on automatic—no magic.

Be sexual and appreciate that part of yourself.

Give love to one special person every day.

Value old friends and always make new ones by being involved, volunteering, joining groups, discussions—book, political, exercise, or other.

Write!—Letters, cards—a daily journal of weather, activities, or feelings.

Enjoy good food, learn to create special dishes for yourself.

Begin early to enhance your own face by appreciating your wisdom and character.

Practice your spiritual beliefs daily by being grateful and positive, even when it seems easier to be negative.

Aging is simply putting in the bank what you hope will be there for you at the end—love and friends.

Feed the animals and birds.

Say your prayers, thank yous, and I love yous often.

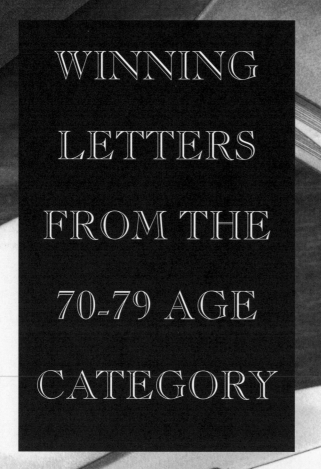

WINNING
LETTERS
FROM THE
70-79 AGE
CATEGORY

James E. Birren

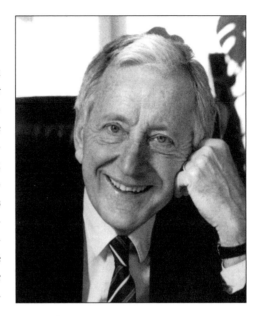

JAMES E. BIRREN, Ph.D., D.Sc., is Associate Director of the UCLA Center on Aging and Professor Emeritus of Gerontology and Psychology at the University of Southern California. His long and distinguished career in the field of gerontology is highlighted by numerous international awards including the Brookdale Foundation Award for Gerontological Research and honorary doctorates from the University of Gothenberg, Sweden, Northwestern University, and St. Thomas University, Canada. Dr. Birren is series editor of the internationally renowned *Handbooks on Aging*, now in their fourth edition, and has over 250 publications in academic journals and books. His most recent publication (1996) is the *Encyclopedia of Gerontology* on which he served as editor-in-chief. Dr. Birren's current book, co-authored with Linda Feldman and to be published by Simon and Schuster, is titled *Where to Go in Your Second Fifty: Discovering the Wisdom of Your Own Life*. The book is about his 20 years of conducting autobiography writing groups here and abroad.

SENIORS OFFER HOPE

Reading these letters gave me hope. Not only for myself, but for all of us and for our country. The writers have built good lives and in their seventies they are optimistic about their futures. They have given us access to the usually inaccessible, to the inside thoughts of elders who know about living long and healthy lives.

These letters describe the important lessons of life the writers have learned. The writers see life clearly and are passing on clues about surviving long and well. They convince me that the strength of America lies in people like these.

In reading these letters one cannot help but be impressed with the wealth of experience and wisdom in our seniors. Their writers are ordinary people on the outside and wise people on the inside as a result of the lessons life has taught them. They have lived through prosperity and depressions, wars and peace, as well as the ups and downs of daily life. We will be greater as a country and as individuals if we listen to them. For this will increase our capacity to manage our own lives better and to manage our country as well.

The young characteristically project on to the old negative stereotyped pictures. Negative atttitudes toward old age lead to dread of growing older rather than the expectation of growing wiser and leading a better life. These letters show that being old in America can be anticipated and appreciated. Clearly, one of the signs of a healthy old age is optimism about tomorrow. In this sense these letter writers convinced me that they are the hope makers of America. Based upon the realism of their life's experiences they have offered us their wisdom. If we respect it, more of us will come to a healthy old age productively, contentedly, and in good health.

These letters support the willingness of the writers to use the freedom their mature lives give them. They have written about what they are doing and what we can do also. They have taught me that they are the hope and the hope makers of America. After reading them I want to do more to help myself lead a healthy life and help myself by helping others. I would like to read more letters like these and try to write some myself.

ALABAMA

William Travis
Age 76
Hoover, AL

Laugh and your heart laughs with you. Robust laughter's target is the whole body; its aim is unconditional joy. Its strikes are relentless. It will not give up. Ever. For whatever ails you, laughter hastens the cure. An encounter with a fit of laughter is surrender to the proper dose of the second best drug in the world, outranked only by love.

No organ, no tissue, no system of the body and lungs can ever escape the rewards of laughter. The brain, blood, and lungs all respond. The skin and bones relish laughter. The eyes; the nose; the digestive tract. Glands are big winners. The immune system rejoices. Hormones are released. Respiration and digestion gain. Pain and depression also gain—their comeuppance.

When you plant cuttings of laughter, the vines and leaves and tendrils will reach out to every part of your body. The fruit is delicious; the harvest plentiful—and your song will harmonize with every fruitful movement.

Absent pain and depression, you will be able to make keen decisions, enjoy fun and games and volunteer activity—laughter's gift to your spirit—and hold to fast the respect of those even younger than you—laughter's reward to your children's spirits.

ALASKA

Harriet Botelho
Age 78
Juneau, AK

The cardinal principle of Healthy Aging is to "keep moving," both mentally and physically.

As a senior, one discovers that although many doors have closed, other opportunities exist to add an exciting dimension to one's life. Decreasing reliance on material possessions enables one to experience the joy of using resources to support worthy causes and help others. Healthy Aging encompasses involvement with people of all ages. This finds expression by volunteering at schools, day care centers, and shelters.

Whatever one's limitations, plan a day that includes some physical activity, a nutritious meal, sufficient rest, and avoidance of stress. Be grateful for what you can do.

Remember it's never too late to learn a new skill—even computers! Participate in an Elderhostel. Laugh heartily often. Practice kindness. Be enthusiastic about something outside your own four walls.

Maintain an avid interest in social/political affairs. Don't hesitate to voice opinions on issues. No one is going to "fire" you for speaking your mind!

Finally, one needs a spiritual bulwark to meet the sorrows, loss, and disappointments that come our way and to face the future with eternal hope.

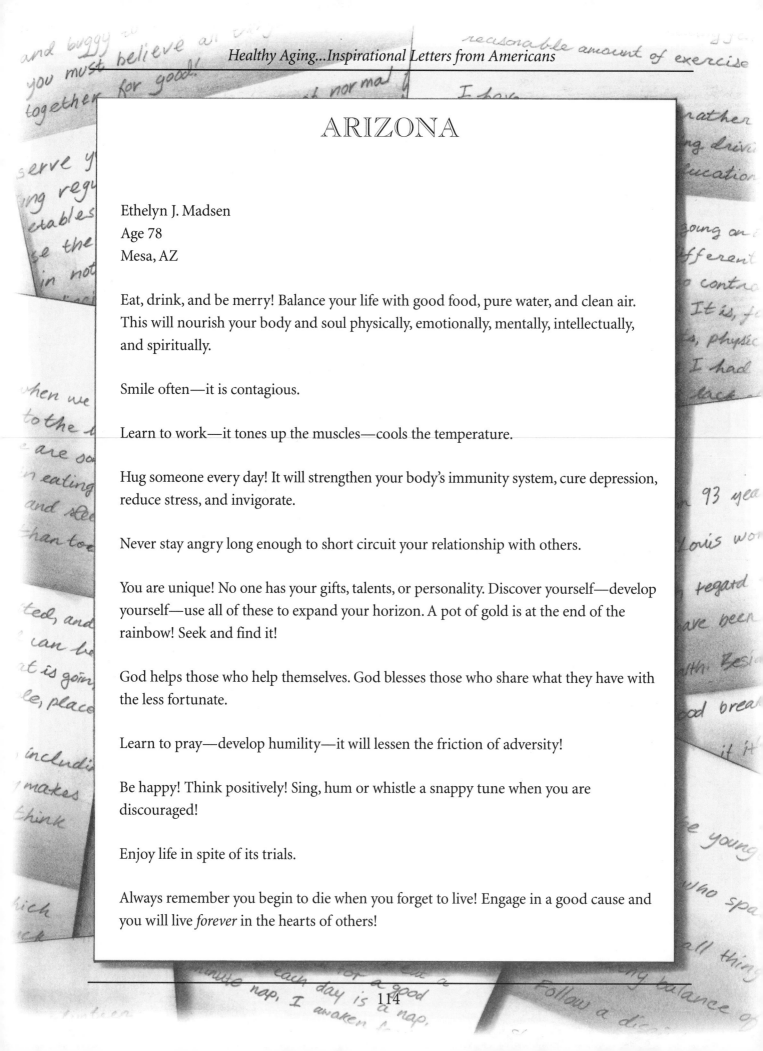

ARIZONA

Ethelyn J. Madsen
Age 78
Mesa, AZ

Eat, drink, and be merry! Balance your life with good food, pure water, and clean air. This will nourish your body and soul physically, emotionally, mentally, intellectually, and spiritually.

Smile often—it is contagious.

Learn to work—it tones up the muscles—cools the temperature.

Hug someone every day! It will strengthen your body's immunity system, cure depression, reduce stress, and invigorate.

Never stay angry long enough to short circuit your relationship with others.

You are unique! No one has your gifts, talents, or personality. Discover yourself—develop yourself—use all of these to expand your horizon. A pot of gold is at the end of the rainbow! Seek and find it!

God helps those who help themselves. God blesses those who share what they have with the less fortunate.

Learn to pray—develop humility—it will lessen the friction of adversity!

Be happy! Think positively! Sing, hum or whistle a snappy tune when you are discouraged!

Enjoy life in spite of its trials.

Always remember you begin to die when you forget to live! Engage in a good cause and you will live *forever* in the hearts of others!

ARKANSAS

Maxine Brittain Stalcup
Age 76
Mountain View, AR

Golden age—and beyond—can be a pleasurable time to work and be happy with family and friends. One must dare to reach out.

I am now a woman alone, a self-taught herbalist in the Arkansas Ozarks. I have found fulfillment in a busy schedule, in mind and health-stretching activities, in home and extensive herb gardens.

My herbs have created a fantastic life for me in making use of talents acquired during family-rearing days: Gardening, writing, painting, photography, lecturing, rock art, entertaining, and creative-food-ways.

But best of all are the hundreds of new friends who came my way each year.

I collect and use Arkansas wild plants, both edible and medicinal. I create and share my original recipes and remedies.

My favorite way to share is in taking groups on salad walks. We hike the creek, woods and gardens, gathering thirty to sixty flowers, weeds, and herbs.

Then, we head for my happy kitchen to create a beautiful, healthful, and delicious salad dinner. Previously prepared herbal desserts tempt the tasters.

This unique learning experience delights men, women, and children.

I am happy. I have shared. I have taught.

Dare to reach out...

CALIFORNIA

Royal L. Craig
Age 74
Huntington Beach, CA

Dear David:

You have finished school and are about to enter into this new business venture with your young friends. May I tell you a story?

The Hindu god, Lord Vishnu invited the demons to a great feast and when they had assembled, he welcomed them, then added these words, "You may eat all this wonderful food, but there is one stipulation. Don't bend your elbows."

The demons looked at the great feast spread before them, and then at Lord Vishnu. They tried eating without bending their elbows, but without success. Finally, in frustration, they said, "You have tricked us by giving us an impossible task." They went away complaining.

Lord Vishnu then invited the saints to the feast and gave them the same stipulation, "Don't bend your elbows."

The saints pondered the puzzle and said, "Lord Vishnu had a purpose in presenting us with this problem and we should discover what it is."

Finally they saw the solution and began to feed each other. They left the feast, happy and full.

My advice to you and your friends, David, is: Don't bend your elbows, reach out and help each other for a long and fulfilling life.

Love,
Dad

COLORADO

Harold L. Hutchinson
Age 78
Olathe, CO

My Golden Age.

Both Mom and Dad lived by the Golden Rule and made sure their kids knew of the benefits gained.

Being the oldest of ten children, I remember occasions when "Do unto others as you would have others do unto you" did not seem to work out as I thought. However, the Golden Rule was a very good guide to pattern my life.

Forming good moral habits is necessary for a healthy, happy life. An orderly life of truthfulness, thoughtfulness, gentleness, industry, punctuality, loving, and respect for our fellow man has to lead to a richer, fuller life.

Doing what is right eliminates the necessity of having to say "I'm sorry."

I indeed feel fortunate to have been given this time to see new advances like refrigeration, automobiles, airplanes, medical progress, television, radio, computers, and space travel.

It has been a "golden age."

CONNECTICUT

Chester W. Harris
Age 76
Waterbury, CT

Dear Younger American:

Does survival of the Great Depression, four wars, several natural disasters, the experiences of being a WW II soldier, a husband, father, and grandfather qualify me as an advisor to you? Perhaps not, but like chicken soup, it shouldn't hurt!

Herewith, then, I offer the following for your consideration:

1. Do not look for great "highs" in drugs but, rather, experience the *real* highs that joyful participation in life itself will bring.

2. Meet all problems as challenges, not obstacles. You *can* mold the kind of life you want.

3. Live in a manner that will allow you to really like yourself.

4. Do not keep your head above water by standing on another's shoulders. Learn to swim.

5. Do not expect life to be "fair." It isn't. Accept good fortune and ill fortune as inevitable experiences of living and allow neither to dominate your life.

6. In good times read "Polonius' Advice to Laertes" from Shakespeare's *Hamlet*.

7. In bad times, read William Ernest Henley's *Invictus*.

8. As you age, add positive concepts to your own philosophy, seeking always integrity, honor, optimism, and love; eschewing negativism, despair, and defeat.

9. Remember that in you rests the immortality of we who proceed you and of the visions we pursued.

Happy and Healthy Aging!

DELAWARE

Helen Day
Age 74
Rehoboth, DE

The single most important thing I have learned about Healthy Aging is love.

The older one gets the more one gets to love life. Every aspect of it. Loving anything keeps one healthy and happy.

I love my husband, children, and grandchildren. They come first. And yes, I even love my in-laws.

How wonderful to work at a job you love and get paid for it. That would keep you on a high for most of your life.

To keep healthy and therefore happy, keep an open mind. Join clubs, volunteer, experience the art, music, and food of other cultures.

I love gardening, needlepoint, crossword puzzles. Keep a dog as a pet. Nothing else will teach you the meaning of unqualified love. I love to travel. I would dearly love to see the whole world before I die.

I love the changing seasons.

Holidays at my house are celebrated with joyous abandon. The whole family comes on the fourth of July. Dresses in red, white, and blue—gets their musical instruments and parades around the block. Christmas is truly a celebration of joy and love. Family, gifts galore, lights, laughter, love of God.

Love! Love! Love! You'll stay young, happy, and surely healthy.

DISTRICT OF COLUMBIA

Ms. Indiana Evans
Age 73
Washington, DC

Dear Future Generations:

I will be 74 years old on December 2, 1996. I want you to be physically healthy like I am when you get to my age, but you may have to make some changes in your lifestyle. I know that I had to make some changes, because I have not always been as healthy as I am now. When I was 53, I had angina so bad that I had to go to the emergency room two or three times a month. I had to put a pill under my tongue to try to control it. I had no restrictions on my diet. I ate everything fried. My older sister ate the same way I did. When she died with a heart attack, I was shocked. I was so frightened.

I went to a nutritionist. I went on a low fat diet. It really worked, because I have not had chest pains in over 20 years.

I have no major health problems now.

I am a retired teacher, but I still work as a substitute teacher. I still take my walks daily. Please get on a low fat diet. Control your future health.

FLORIDA

Irving Shavelson
Age 77
Coconut Creek, FL

Healthy Aging? How can you dare to be sick when you have 100 or so children waiting for you to read stories to them, sing songs with them, and entertain them with magic tricks?

On retiring to Florida, I volunteered to read to children of pre-kindergarten age in a program sponsored by the library system. I now read four days each week, two days at the library and two days at local day schools.

How can one feel old when surrounded by beautiful young children? I look up from my reading on some days and look at those lovely faces, eyes open in wonderment at the tales that I am reading or telling. By the end of the session I feel ten years younger!

At one program my subject was "what do you want to be when you grow up?" One child hesitated when I asked her the question. "Don't worry," I told her, "I am 77 years old and I still don't know what I want to be when I grow up." "Yes," she responded, "but you're already up." She was right.

I was really up, up in the air from such wonderful experiences.

GEORGIA

Teresa Rigby
Age 76
Dunwoody, GA

Why be lonely?

There is an exciting world out there with people like you waiting for a contact. Write that friend of old or send a card.

Travel! Send for free brochures, find the one you would like to go to, get a video from the library, and sit back and enjoy. If you don't have a video, sit back and dream.

Enter free contests; one never knows, you could be a winner, it's the excitement it brings. Send for free samples. The papers and grocery stores always have them, on shelves and boards. Then there are do it yourself brochures, yours for the sending of a card or letter.

Having a bad day—everything is going wrong, feeling sorry for yourself—write all that is bothering you down, put in envelope, and address it to yourself. A few days later when it arrives you will see how foolish it was for today is the opposite.

Keep those letters going and coming. The postman is your best friend.

HAWAII

Hope Dennis
Age 77
Laie, HI

As Young As I Wanna Be

Please don't be taken in
by this old lady mask
I wear.

Look into my eyes,

Please.

And see me.

Still sixteen

Still at the dance
and with a jumprope
still clutched in one hand.

IDAHO

Eldon H. Mattson
Age 78
St. Charles, ID

Gettin' Old

What it's all about, you'll never guess.

How to stay young, and still grow old.

This is a story that's never been told.

Inspire others to live a good healthy life—

In this mixed up world of toil and strife.

Stay alert when driving or you may get hit.

Avoid vicious dogs or you may get bit.

Stay away from drugs or you'll get hooked.

Keep out of trouble or you'll get booked.

Don't drink and drive, better still, just don't drink.

Your head will stay clear when you need to think.

Smoking's not smart—it's really so sad

To clog up your lungs that you need so bad.

Select good foods to eat every day;

Remember the slogan—"an apple a day."

Don't shy away from work—it's the best exercise.

Get up early each day to see the sun rise.

Be kind and good to your wife—and be *true*.

She will be your best friend and sweetheart too.

In seventy eight years I may not know the score—

But I'm happy and healthy and hoping for more.

ILLINOIS

Frances Hawley
Age 75
Odin, IL

A New Love in My Life.

Jessica, the grandchild that God did not deem it possible for me to have. Jessica, the gift that God sent to me to take my husband's place.

When my husband died in 1992, I was faced with the realization that I would forever be alone. I was 71 years old and since age 31 had been afflicted with scoliosis and arthritis of the spine. Through the years, I swam for therapy and also taught over 200 children to swim.

Three days after my husband's funeral, I was asked to teach a five-year-old to swim. Thus, Jessica came into my life. Each Friday, I would meet her at the Holidome in Mt. Vernon and she would put her arms around my neck and say "I love you."

Jessica is now nine years old and has broken many swim records throughout Southern Illinois.

I still miss my husband, but I find happiness in the hours I spend with Jessica and fulfillment in the knowledge that the many children I have taught to swim will practice water safety. At age 75, I exercise and swim daily and look forward to the future when Jessica will be an Olympic Champion.

INDIANA

Ruth S. Lambert
Age 75
Crown Point, IN

Healthy Aging doesn't just happen! It is acquired by living every day, a day at a time to your utmost ability.

I grew up during the Great Depression. We couldn't waste anything. Everything was appreciated and had to be used. World War II followed graduation from high school. All things were rationed—cars, gasoline, food, soap, even stockings and shoes. We learned to go without extras so our soldiers had amenities, food, and warm clothing. We gave up freely—sometimes grumbling, but proud to support our men and country. Families "doubled up" as manpower and lumber for housing just wasn't available. We prayed too—did we pray!! Afterward everyone worked to rebuild our personal lives, overcome loss of friends, sons, fathers, and husbands. Those were the greatest losses!

Unless future generations learn the very difficult lessons of life—the spirit of giving and the inspiration and work to rebuild after difficulties, to go forward with love and devotion to God and fellow men, to build a better world, we'll not promote financial responsibility, physical, social, and mental well-being. Emotional and Healthy Aging will not be achieved without spirit that promotes love of others and physical and mental well-being.

IOWA

Marion S. Clark
Age 72
Cedar Falls, IA

Dear Child of the Future:

If I have learned anything, it is that *we* are the drum major in our parade of life.

There is so much health information out there, sometimes it's so overwhelming that we would like to chuck it all and do as we please.

But if you weigh the information, decide what you can live with, and make some good decisions, you're going to have a good quality of life. It may not be longer, but you will feel better.

In my lifetime there have been amazing medical discoveries—insulin and penicillin to name two. The discoveries in your lifetime will be even more surprising and spectacular, hopefully a cure for cancer.

So for now, eat your carrots, drink your milk, take your vitamins, eat fiber, exercise, and *keep informed*. The rules change constantly, and you are the one who has to stay current.

Oh, I forgot to mention not to abuse smoking, drugs, and alcohol (just had to bring those up!). Get involved in these and you'll be huffing, puffing, and staggering as you try to lead your parade. Some drum major you'll be!

Love from a health nut.

KANSAS

Katherine F. Penner
Age 77
Inman, KS

It is not what happens to us, but how we handle it that matters. Consider each day a gift from God. It has been proven that a positive attitude helps prevent and heal illnesses. "A merry heart doeth good like medicine." Proverbs 17:22.

Diet is not a dirty, four-letter word. A healthy diet consisting of vegetables, fruit, and a minimal amount of meat does much to keep your body strong and youthful.

Exercise in the morning to make the day go well. Beautiful sunrises, birds singing, invigorating fresh air to fill the lungs—these are rewards for getting up early.

Much grief and unhappiness can be prevented by avoiding tobacco, drugs, alcohol, and illicit sex. Cigarettes are killers that travel in packs. If you must drink, drink water—eight glasses a day is the recommended amount.

Mountain climbing over molehills can produce ulcers. Sometimes wanting less is greater riches than having more.

A day wrapped in prayer is less likely to unravel. Fear not the future. The great Creator is still in control and He cares for you . Miracles still happen and God does answer prayers.

KENTUCKY

Betty Brawner
Age 79
Louisville, KY

Be Happy.

Helen Keller said, "Many persons have the wrong idea of what constitutes happiness. It is not attained through self-gratitude but through fidelity to a worthy purpose."

I am thankful for the wisdom to realize that I could not change the world around me. But I changed *my* world settings—the world I make and control. By changing my reactions and attitudes, the world at large responds more positively with me.

Many people seem to expect life to react abundantly toward them without so much as investing anything in the way of time, effort, or prayer. Many people ask the earth to feed them. Ancient wisdom says till the soil, plant the seed, nourish them, and keep out the intrusive life-sapping weeds. The earth will repay you.

We are imperfect people living in an imperfect world. We must accept evil as part of life; a fact of life. Be realistic and hopeful. God is not dead nor does He sleep. The wrong shall fail; the right prevail with peace on earth, good will toward men.

Positive attitude is most important. See the good in others. There is some good in everyone.

LOUISIANA

Pierre V. Daigle
Age 72
Church Point, LA

After living 72 years, I see the following concepts and principles as the key to Healthy Aging.

1. Don't wait until you're old to prepare! Education, knowledge, and awareness add to life's scope and flavors!

2. Keep learning. Learn by reading, by studying, by listening, by observing, by *doing*! Teach others. It's a great way to learn!

3. Work hard, be honest: Work doesn't kill; a bad conscience can.

4. Shun delusions. It takes more guts to stay with a spouse, raise children, face the daily grind—than it does to bungee jump.

5. Never forget that life is meant to be a search for flavors: in cooking, in living, in sex. Love of life is the master flavor.

6. Marriage is meant to be an ever-widening circle of teaching and learning. A man learns from his wife. He takes what she teaches, makes it better, teaches the wider circle back to her. She enlarges it, passes it back to him. By the time their circle is half as large as life is meant to be, their time is over. No time for boredom. No chauvinist guilt; no rancor of feminism!

MAINE

Jeannette S. Cross
Age 71
Brunswick, ME

Some of us have good health as our special blessing in retirement. How to hold onto that advantage is a challenge. For me this means celebration with food—making its preparation and presentation a meaningful art form that feeds the soul as it nourishes the body. While following this path brings great rewards to the mental and physical self (I was born to cook!) it touches happily the lives of those around me. Feeding others with care is a form of loving that is welcomed wherever it comes to rest. Comfort and feeling well fed, with a body that will do what you ask of it, are real goals. In the process of pursuing this reality daily, there is heightened adventure: Meeting people, walking to shop, gardening, composting, sharing recipes and reading what is happening in the field of nutrition, and using yourself, your family, and your friends as your private research and experimentation program. Each of us is empowered to give. The tools for me are in the kitchen, and the celebration is at the table where happiness is.

MARYLAND

Marcia Potter
Age 71
Easton, MD

Finally Senior! A royal rank I had dreamed of through protracted progression...Fearful Freshman, Submissive Sophomore, Jaunty Junior, then...Ta Da! Supreme Senior! Pomp and Circumstance down the aisle, tassel swaying...graduation! "Hello world! Here I come!"

Just what *have* I become? Another "graduated" senior...an appetizer at age 50, soup added at 55, the entire menu at 65. Fully aged, ripened, and ready.

Ready for what? *Not* the Depressed Downers Club. "Wait until I'm gone and then..." or "If I'm still here next year..." Don't nudge me toward Finality. The Friendlier Future still beckons.

Shall I join the Poker Game of Ailments? "*You* have arthritis? *I* have arthritis and I'll raise you two bunions!" No winning hands at *that* table!

My winning hand embraces ageless rules:

1. Laugh *at* myself, laugh *with* others.
2. Cherish memories, but seek the new.
3. Foster friendships with care, comfort, and trust.
4. Harbor hope, deny despair.
5. Heed healthy guidelines, but enjoy a chocolate.

True, life is *not* a card game, but I deal not with a stacked deck, but with a rainbow-hued assortment, offering the freedom to shuffle, choose, and savor each hand labeled "Senior."

MASSACHUSETTS

Elin Anderson
Age 79
Dudley, MA

On the threshold of 80, I find myself happy, healthy, and in great shape.

Age doesn't matter—what you do with your life does!

Exercise and love of humanity has been my salvation. I walk the six miles for the CROP walk to feed the hungry. Saw the need to exercise for the elderly, and now run two classes a week. Excellent for health—for mind, body and spirit.

Never set a mental age when you feel you will be old—for when you get there you will be old. Genesis says our bodies were made to last 120 years—so that's when I'll die. God gave us a perfect body—if man made it, it would last 20 years!

Hobbies make life interesting—mine are oil painting, tennis, tai chi, and performing in plays.

I was born poor—still am—but not in spirit! I accept reality and live for now. I love to make people laugh—it's better than medicine.

I consider it a privilege to be part of creation!

MICHIGAN

David C. Freshel
Age 71
Allen Park, MI

Healthy Aging: Learning from the Trees.

It ain't what you don't know, that does the harm:
It's what you do know, that ain't so.

Early American Humorist

As I approach my 73rd year, I'm grateful to have spent the last 30 as a tree doctor.

These trees, some of which I've known for more than a quarter century, have questioned me on a deeply-instilled conceptual error, by which I've been misguided:

Why do [they]—a species at the zenith of the vegetable kingdom—grow larger and stronger with age, and can survive centuries or millennia...while [I]—purportedly at the zenith of the animal kingdom and created in the image and likeness of God—expect to shrink, weaken, and die?

It becomes clearer to me that my problems stem not from divine design but from adverse, self-fulfilling prophecy.

The more I emulate my tree friends in simple acceptance of God's gifts, the bigger, better, and more secure I become.

MINNESOTA

Allen (Al) Sandvik
Age 71
Edina, MN

Dear Future Generations of America:

Hello. I thought I'd drop you a line.
From up here on the mountain.
At 71, I'm near the end of the climb.

I look back at those who are steadily elevating, day by day getting somewhere. But then so many are going around, sometimes down, the mountain; not realizing or caring that their life is being spent for nothing.

Me, I wanted to be a writer. So I found myself a job as office boy in a large advertising agency. In time I moved to another agency, and years of work later, became its president.

A friend of mine wrote a book called *If You Don't Know Where You're Going, How Will You Know When You Get There?*

Even if you are in the foothills, let your mind take hold of the whole of the mountain. Understand there's somewhere for you to go, something for you to give. Then take your first step in that direction.

If you stay with it, the trek of aging will have more and more meaning at every station. Achieving is one of the best ways I know to be alive, from start to finish.

MISSISSIPPI

Jason N. Kutack
Age 71
Hattiesburg, MS

My Grandchildren:

To age healthy, observe the following:

Worship a higher power. Obey the 10 commandments for spiritual survival.

Perfect your reading skills. With them you can gain the equivalent of a college education.

Form the habit of saving 10% of all you earn. With the magic of compound interest, you will maintain independence.

Take care of your body with good diet, exercise, and sleep. Eschew drugs, alcohol, and tobacco; they kill.

Be a friend to make friends. No man is an island.

Serve your community, whether in the services, a professional, a politician, an activist, or a voter. This strengthens our democracy.

Have a family, traditional or not, to foster and care for. This makes life exciting and worthwhile, enabling human society to progress and improve.

Finally, when you realize your talents and abilities and recognize your dreams, bolster your courage to risk to achieve them.

Then, in the autumn of your life, in retirement you will have the satisfaction of knowing that your efforts and sacrifices were worthy.

MISSOURI

Richard F. Ferguson
Age 76
Carthage, MO

A Letter to Future Generations:

Healthy Aging, as I am experiencing my time in this 20th century, can be adapted by others, their peers and contemporaries, now and in the future.

Physically, there is a need to take care of and fine tune one's body. At age 15, I was on a state championship cross country team; today, I walk two miles in 30 minutes.

Socially, the art of conversation is a must. Learn the language, speak it with the acuity of an expert. In 1958, I suffered no loss of words when introduced to former President Harry S. Truman. Be enthusiastic!

Mentally, honest self-esteem and a good attitude are commendable, but one does not always have to be politically correct. Admire those whom you would emulate and exude confidence piggybacked by good manners. Set goals.

Financially, a person does not have to "live high off the hog" to enjoy the good life; there are opportunities, rewards, challenges, and beautiful sunsets out there. Time is your most precious possession, yet it is too soon gone. Save something for your own sunset years.

Keep in touch with Mom and Dad, siblings, and others. Be a leader, acknowledge first class postage as a communications bargain!

MONTANA

Doris Whithorn
Age 79
Livingston, MT

Dear Future Generation:

Here are 10 Commandments for Healthy Aging:

1. Remember each day that all you need to be truly happy is something to be enthusiastic about.

2. Thou shalt exercise moderation in all things—food, drink, spending, accumulation of worldly goods.

3. Get some exercise but also plenty of rest.

4. Stay close to your family, never criticizing during an open confrontation. Write them your reproof and consider it long and with love before giving it wings, whether to them or the wastebasket.

5. Cultivate younger friends, but do not burden them with stories of your youth, unless asked.

6. Thou shalt let your conscience be your guide in questionable situations.

7. Do something nice for someone each day and let someone do something special for you.

8. Express appreciation for even small favors that you may be considered grateful.

9. Thou shalt read something inspirational daily to find, for instance, in a poem, word pictures to be painted on the soul; in proverbs, how to be content with your own life; in a mystery story, excitement to dream of.

10. Dwell not on your infirmities, but prepare for the inevitable.

NEBRASKA

Donald Cushenbery
Age 71
Omaha, NE

Regardless of age, race, color, or income, every human being will experience grief and hurt. When you encounter loss, there are at least two aspects that you should remember. First, there are many situations which should befall you over which you can't control. Second, when you are hurting, don't dwell on the negative parts of the problem and become defeated. Turn a lemon into lemonade. My wife of 37 years died in 1988 after a long illness. Because of her death, I was inspired to co-author a widely read book to help others who have lost a mate. *Remember*: It is not so important what happens to you...it is *how you react* to what has come your way.

To cope with loss, look forward, not backward. Many individuals live miserable lives because they regret what happened yesterday and fear what might happen tomorrow. Connect with a network of friends and loved ones and let them help you gain strength and comfort from their words, thoughts, and prayers. Emphasize the positives of your life and rise each morning determined with God's help to meet the challenges that may confront you.

NEVADA

Len Hughes
Age 73
Carson City, NV

When I think of Healthy Aging, I thing of Sophie, that tiny, wise, village music teacher who also taught simple secrets for happy living!

Sophie was in her 80s when we first met. She had lost a son and twice been widowed, yet she was so at ease with her world...

One morning, as I started to rush off to whatever the day held, I felt Sophie's hand in gentle restraint. "Let me say something," she cautioned.

"You are robust because you follow sensible hygiene rules. You enjoy a balanced diet, and you get enough sleep and exercise. But, you could gain more from life.

"Each day, before you enter the lists, pause a moment. Put everything else out of mind, and concentrate on activities that bring greatest satisfaction. A fresh mindset instills a sense of well-being—and then the body works wonders!"

I tried. Of course it worked, for everything originates in the mind.

Did Sophie practice her own "mindset" philosophy? Evidently. On her 90th birthday she played piano and sang for guests. Everyone applauded as she hit all the high notes in her rendition of "I'm the Happiest Girl in the Whole USA!"

NEW HAMPSHIRE

Mary M. Wyman
Age 79
Concord, NH

How do we make the next generation responsive to ours and live healthy lives? We who have survived want to pass on the wisdom gained by our attention to proper nutrition and exercise.

I wanted a college education but circumstances and the Depression prevented it after high school. I felt the lack. It resulted in my seeking knowledge. Eventually it led to the opportunity to take college courses. Over the years I accumulated credits and on my 70th birthday I was awarded a degree. The pursuit sustained me over the years through many difficult situations and taught me how to cope. It is said that using the mind preserves it. One is never too old to learn. It is a lifetime experience and keeps one healthy.

Because I missed going to college when I was young, it taught me the value of learning, it kept my curiosity alive; it taught me to choose what was best and make choices and act upon them. This resulted in keeping a healthy attitude.

I am a target archer, and as someone once said, "The song I came to sing remains unsung, but I continue to string and unstring my bow."

NEW JERSEY

Arthur Zirul
Age 72
Fairview, NJ

Who are these frenzied seniors I read about? Octogenarians who fly jet planes? Septuagenarians who risk their lives climbing high mountains? And the most incredible seniors of all—those who want to continue working until they drop? I know none of these people.

The seniors I know are all rational beings who enjoy aging at a leisurely, healthy pace. After a lifetime of hard work, my friends and I looked forward to a retirement filled with simple pleasures. Face it, most of us did not "love" our jobs. What we did love was getting away from those jobs on weekends and vacations. Well, retirement is an endless vacation. We would have to be crazy to jeopardize that by risking our health in harmful pursuits.

We would rather play cards than fly airplanes. We prefer checkers to climbing mountains, and gentle strolls to endless labor. It's not challenging? It's not rewarding? Nonsense. What's challenging or rewarding about risking injury or, even worse, dying on the job?

The best way to Healthy Aging is to age gracefully. Think cool, think calm, think smelling the roses. Think about enjoying the simple things in life.

NEW MEXICO

Hal Shymkus
Age 70
Espanola, NM

Too often senior people put off fulfilling a lifelong ambition by saying, "Oh, I wouldn't be any good doing that."

In my opinion, that comment is humbuggery. Anyone can do what they want to do if they only set their mind to it.

After attending a concert at the Senior Center, a woman says, "I've always wanted to play the piano." A retired business executive, after reading a marketing book, reflects, "Why, I could write a book on that subject."

Well, do it! Take lessons. Make the effort.

You may not play like Van Cliburn or write like Steven R. Covey but you will be surprised how accomplished you can become and how personally rewarding the outcome will be.

I always wanted to write and began doing so upon retirement at age 60. In the past ten years I have had published over 100 fiction and non-fiction pieces as well as two books.

I am proud and pleased at what I have done. And there is so much more writing ahead. Had I not made the effort and stayed with it, I would not be writing this letter.

NEW YORK

Jess C. Weston
Age 72
Long Beach, NY

Young America, I urge you to go beyond routine conventional dietary regimens, appropriate exercising efforts, required immunizations, recommended medical and dental checkups, and the avoidance of ingesting harmful substances by incorporating into your daily life the planning of pleasurable future activities.

Always have something to look forward to. If you like to travel, plan your trip well in advance. Theater, music, dance, sporting events, or any other diversion of your taste should be scheduled by you, for you at a reasonable foreseeable date. Some pliability must be accommodated according to your specific living conditions, but a plan must be in place.

Simply always have something "going for you" that entails some planning and preparation and discussion with a partner to ensure the best possible experiences. Enjoy your time, but keep part of your mind on what you can make happen!

NORTH CAROLINA

Rodney D. Steinmetz, M.D.
Age 71
Fleetwood, NC

As a 71-year-old male with a family history of heart disease, I try to maintain a healthy lifestyle including aerobic exercise, weight training, stretching, and a low fat nutritious diet.

When we retired to a rural area, I wanted to contribute to the community. Some Swiss Olympic athletes had stated that they liked our country except for the litter on our beautiful roads. Motivated by that information I "adopted" five miles of a country road where I run regularly. After the initial clean-up, I found that I could easily patrol the area twice a week when doing my daily three-mile runs. My heart monitor indicates that stopping to pick up a piece of litter does not significantly affect my pulse rate, so I am still getting the aerobic exercise I need.

An unexpected bonus is the response from local residents. Many people have stopped to say how much they appreciate my efforts.

When using proper safety and healthy precautions, adopting a road can be a healthy, satisfying experience for anyone, regardless of age, who enjoys walking or running.

NORTH DAKOTA

Alda C. Sobak
Age 72
Edmore, ND

Society is so conscious of age. It stresses age as it relates to calendar years rather than to the continuous development of soul, mind, and talents.

Healthy Aging is demonstrated by an invalid gathering youngsters close at eventide to point out the galaxies in the night sky; or by a retired teacher volunteering time and energy to tutor immigrants; by a musician subduing pain to teach and enthrall wide-eyed listeners. A grandmother, recovering from by-pass surgery, from memory, accompanies the choir at Sunday services.

Not giving up the exercising of mind, body, and talents, but passing on the wonders of life to younger, eager open minds, and hearts—this is Healthy Aging.

How to accomplish this?

First, greet each day with praise and thanksgiving for life, for people, for a world of indescribable wonders, above all for a forgiving savior.

Second, treat your body as a holy temple. Fill mind and heart with love, kindness, understanding, and forgiveness.

Third, accept your limitations, but use your days and years for service to others; whether it be family, friends, or strangers. Thus by giving of oneself with joy, we experience healthy living.

OHIO

Eleanor W. Schmidt
Age 78
Columbiana, OH

My Grandmother (Catherine Louisa Baughman Jewel 1860-1937) took me to visit her friends at the old ladies home*. Her instructions to an eight-year-old, "Sit on a chair and listen. *Remember you will be old someday.*"

Mother (Helen Louise Jewell Wietelmann 1893-1989) encouraged me to always keep my hands busy, even when not feeling well.

Sunday afternoons I spend visiting residents without company at Parkside Health Care Center*.

Among recent visits:

-The new 62-year-old resident who depressingly said, "I'll be here the rest of my life. My children have sold all my furniture and home."

-The 93-year-old gentleman said, "I was raised by grandparents on a Tennessee farm, I didn't go to school, I had chores, loved to fish, and work in the garden." He is a World War I veteran.

-The resident who constantly crochets beautiful afghans in spite of her arthritic gnarled fingers.

A resident's son said to me, "It's so nice of you to visit, cheering them up with your pleasant smile."

I return to my apartment, count my many blessings, and after 78 years say a prayer of appreciation for lessons taught a child.

*Old Ladies Home, now an historical site. Woodlawn Ave., Zanesville, OH
*Parkside Health Care Center, 930 E. Park Ave., Columbiana, OH

OKLAHOMA

Joseph W. Dean
Age 76
Idabel, OK

At age 75 I was asked to retire as pastor of our country church. "Yes! Willingly! To provide an opportunity for a younger man!"

Then I offered my services to the neighboring parish. The pastor was happy to obtain an assistant because he was serving both an English speaking and a Spanish speaking community! To become more useful I decided to learn Spanish. It would be a stimulating challenge!

To make such study worthwhile, one should figure at least 15 years of service. So I determined to stay healthy for 15 more years.

During the past year this experience of learning Spanish, of shepherding a new kind of congregation, of looking forward to continuing actively, has triggered a new source of energy and enthusiasm. Now I have motivation to watch my diet, take daily walks, and stay young at heart.

Social and financial health were automatically taken care of. The people appreciate my efforts so much that they provide food, clothing, even recreation that I never expected! I am excited to experience that in giving you do receive and in loving you are loved. I have learned that you can't spread happiness around without spilling some on yourself.

OREGON

Alice Gillenwater
Age 71
Bend, OR

Dear Glen:

Today my best friend, counselor, comforter passed away. An accident with a loaded cement truck and pickup at a highway crossing necessitated air flight to the hospital, x-rays, intensive care, and respiratory assistance. He suffered five fractured ribs, severe bruises over back and arms and probably undiscovered injuries. Although initial prognosis was guarded, I prayed that he would recover.

Ironic, it was his lungs that took his life after twelve days, just short of seventy years. Smoking since a teenager, he unsuccessfully tried to quit several times, managing to curtail it half in recent months.

This morning 9:00 A.M. Denise called—Doctor had advised that John's condition was deteriorating. At his bedside we massaged his extremities, adjusted the pillow/sheets trying to make him more comfortable and simultaneously bolstering our courage and grief. He appeared to be sleeping soundly with little recognition of our presence. But the end came four hours later, peacefully (as the doctor said it would). He could *no longer expel the used air* from his lungs.

Are you still smoking?

PENNSYLVANIA

Ellen Feeley
Age 72
Windber, PA

When my husband and I were young parents a widowed neighbor told us how her dreams of traveling were thwarted because she and her husband had "put off" traveling until his retirement. Her husband died, her health failed, and their dreams dissolved—never to come true.

We took her story to heart. We, too, loved to travel. With our two sons, we made plans and we traveled as much and as far as we could.

And now as a healthy, aging widow many of my travel dreams have happened and been shared with those I loved.

For Healthy Aging, turn your dreams into memories long before you reach retirement. Then, with faith, financial resources, and a bit of luck you will be free to create new dreams.

RHODE ISLAND

Anita C. Petrucci
Age 77
North Providence, RI

Healthy aging brings with it the freedom of choice. I had done all the things expected of a woman of my era.

I had borne two sets of children with a ten year span in-between.

In that ten years I had enjoyed "home and hearth" so thoroughly in my family of six, I did not venture further.

I read incessantly all of the books my children brought home. From psychology, anthropology, sociology, physiology, nursing, law enforcement, and "what have you?"

With my neighbor I took many courses in theology.

At 52 years of age I decided to take some serious courses and I obtained a position tutoring under-achievers at two elementary schools in my town. I learned to drive for this endeavor. My daughter gave me her Corvair convertible and I was all on my own.

My husband felt threatened but later made me gourmet lunches on his days off.

He realized I had to prove to myself I was more than a housewife and mother.

Later still, I began writing and still am.

You can have it all and give yourself an entity. An identity. Especially after 50. I did.

SOUTH CAROLINA

Lincoln D. Moody
Age 78
Garden City Beach, SC

The older I grow, the more often I experience the loss of a friend. It makes me sad and remorseful when I realize that I have missed the chance to say "good-bye." It gives me a hollow, achy feeling inside. If I could, I'd call them back to tell them what I wish I'd told them long ago.

So now, whenever my wife or kids or friends leave our house to go in any of a dozen directions, I go to the door and give them a kiss, or a hug, or a kind word as they depart. And I stand there waiting and watching them pull away in their car or walking out of sight. And if they know me, they will turn and glance back knowing I will be standing there. And they will wave and return a kiss, being happy in knowing that if something prevents us from seeing each other again, we will have said our farewell with a glance of friendship or a heart brimming with love. The good feeling will last a lifetime—or until we meet again.

SOUTH DAKOTA

Leo J. Neifer
Age 72
Roscoe, SD

A skinny, virile man of 72 is what my partner has. At fifty years, I viewed my age group; the double chins, round bellies, and floppy thighs urged me avoid what I saw around me.

Observing and reading, I learned the lesson for the balance of my life, namely, that Healthy Aging required a health war against time. Time will win, finally, but it wins sooner with allies foolishly provided with the unhealthy foods we love to eat.

I formed an army: first, a squad of chickens, armed with fat-free stuffing, destroyed the frozen dinners, traitors masking as healthy.

My Cereal and Fruit Company captured the entire Egg and Bacon Battalion. Fat-laden meat products fell to my flotilla fish dishes, prepared with olive oil, a tad of lemon, and spices.

Against the Sodium Division, I sent my veteran Flavor Group, spices battle-tested in taste tests. Gratified because salt no longer masks the natural, varied flavors of my Vegetable Division, I won the Protein Medal!

By studying food labels as if a skull and cross bones lurked in each package, I attacked the food industry, time's ally against my Healthy Aging.

TENNESSEE

Theda B. Wells
Age 77
Germantown, TN

In the country school that I attended when I was six, there were three big signs on the wall:

1. Silence is Golden. My teacher said, "in silence you can hear nature speak." She took us walking along the river to hear the rippling water sing. We listened to the humming birds sing as they flitted from flower to flower.

2. Early to Bed, Early to Rise, Makes a Man Healthy, Wealthy, and Wise. Desiring the latter three, I practiced the first two. A restful night caused me to wake refreshed, ready to meet the challenges of each day. I was a wife for 55 years; mother to an adopted daughter, birth mother to two sons and a daughter; mother to 73 foster children; grandmother to 10 grandchildren. Early rising made time for quiet devotion, duties, hobbies, outings, PTA meetings, church activities, and volunteering.

3. Good Listeners Make Good Learners. My teacher explained that good grades depend on listening well to instructions. Wanting good grades, I listened.

Applying these rules to my daily life made possible most material things I envisioned. Now, I volunteer twice a month at my granddaughter's high school. *Life is good*.

TEXAS

June Nelson
Age 73
Donna, TX

Dear Future Partners:

I like to compare my square dance experience to the secret of Healthy Aging.

The most important secret is listen to your caller. I think of God as my caller. The second secret is don't forget to smile. Are you ready? Please be my partner.

Circle Left. Square dancing is friendship set to music, so join hands with the world around you, concentrate on the needs of others, and share your many blessings.

Grand Square. Here is your chance to participate in the grand square of life. Listen to the caller. Hear him call—work hard, play hard, laugh often, and share your joys and sorrows.

Chase Right. You will meet many leaders in your dance of life. Choose your mentors carefully and learn from them.

Track Two. We all get on the wrong track sometimes and disrupt the square. Here we learn to forgive and be forgiven. Square up your set. Listen to your caller and get back on the right track.

Promenade Home. Just as you complete the circle of life, so the square dance is complete as you join your hands in the final words of thanksgiving and commitment.

I wave to you across the square.

UTAH

Ray L. Bergman
Age 78
Midvale, UT

To Friends Turning Fifty:

If your secret passion is donning black leather and riding byways on a motorcycle, you have the choice. Do it!

If you imagine yourself dancing on your toes, do it! Throw off inhibitions that keep you from realizing your potential and your physical and mental health.

Don't worry about censoring from family members who criticize your audacity.

Don't let religious conventions or fear of unknown perils confound you.

Take advice from a senior of 78. Chart your future now despite minor health problems that nag.

I've attended 38 senior programs through wonderful Elderhostel—over a hundred classes on subjects ranging from Andrew Lloyd Webber's music; history of the Universe; Yoga; to Shakespeare's tragedies.

I was inspired by a wheelchair-bound lady attending Hidden Valley ballet class and doing only arm movements, but enjoying her share of the group experience. Her positive attitude guaranteed a happy success.

Healthy Aging is learning new things despite handicaps; reading books, including Braille; listening even if by lip-reading; enjoying art and the theater; experiencing new places; taking classes.

From "Healthy Aging," the Fountain of Youth "resides in each of us, waiting to be released by the choices we make."

VERMONT

George E. Philcox
Age 74
Plainfield, VT

To You of the Future Generation:

As I now accept the fact that I am old, one thing becomes increasingly clear to me: one of the most important ways to stay young in mind, spirit, and even in body is to be able to laugh. There is no better medicine. The ability to laugh with someone, to make someone laugh, and most important, to be able to laugh at yourself, will get you through the traumas and sorrows of living.

There is almost nothing so terrible or so sad in life that does not have some small (often large) element of humor in it. Laughter makes the medicine work better, laughter makes the pain easier to bear; laughter makes people like you and brings them closer; laughter lets you put the overwhelming into perspective and makes a solution easier.

It matters little whether people laugh at you or with you for the laughter makes life easier, interesting, and not to be overlooked, *Fun*! One giggle, one smile, one good laugh is better than a barrel of tears.

VIRGINIA

Peggy Dwyier
Age 76
Woodstock, VA

Simple prescription for Healthy Aging: *Never be bored.*

How do I avoid boredom?

During the growing season, I garden for a couple of hours in the morning on our beautiful farm in the Shenandoah Valley of Virginia. We bought it 15 years ago when I was 61 and my husband was 62. After gardening, I dress and head for the office of a company I helped to start 48 years ago. As I drive I am aware of my surroundings; the sunrise, the mists above the river, blue mountains, leaves, fresh minted in spring and ablaze with color in the fall. At the office, there is no time for boredom. Psychic income from grateful clients is more important now than when I was young.

Financial concerns? Our tastes are very simple. Money saved during earlier years is sufficient for our needs.

Often, we have the company of a grandchild or two. They are an endless source of fascination for us. In our woods is a picnic table (put there by the gnomes)...there's a hollow tree where the children are quite certain the woodland folks live.

How could I not be a healthy elder with all of this to live for! My cup runneth over.

WASHINGTON

Mary E. Brown
Age 79
Enumclaw, WA

My Dearest Grandson:

Remember how eager you were to be "old enough" to go to kindergarten? How excited you were when you were "old enough" to play soccer?

Because I'll be 80 on my next birthday, you may think I'm beyond being "old enough" for anything.

But I'm not "old enough" to stop learning new things, so I'm trying new tricks—like how to do a spread sheet on my computer to keep track of my medical records.

And I'm not "old enough" to stop admiring all the wonderful things in the world around me—like the total eclipse of the moon last month.

"Old enough" has nothing to do with waiting till some time in the future to be helpful to others and your community. I keep an updated calendar of arts events, run off copies, and distribute them around town.

I'll never be "old enough" to stop loving and being loved—as you and I love each other. I just hope I'll be "old enough" to set foot in the 21st century and see you grow up to be a man.

In fact, I think I'll never again wait to be "old enough." I know you won't either.

WEST VIRGINIA

Anita D. Brown
Age 72
Harpers Ferry, WV

Romance Begins at Seventy!

That's my kind of headline. The lesson learned is that it's never too late to follow a dream.

All my life I yearned to become a writer like Mary Stewart, Pearl Buck, and Phyllis Whitney. Too busy raising three children and working full time, I realized my dream was an impractical fantasy. Maybe, some day...

The children grew up, were educated, left home. I lost a parent, then my mother developed Parkinson's Disease. While caring for her, I had medical problems of my own.

Now in my sixties, was it too late to make my dreams come true? I studied. I wrote. My work was often rejected, but it wasn't a fatal experience. I went on.

Five years later, on my 70th birthday, my first published full-length romance novel arrived. It's not a huge book and it doesn't have a hard cover. I love it!

Four published novels later, I plan to write well into my 80s. When Romance strikes, it doesn't matter that you're 70-something!

WISCONSIN

Harold A. Vanselow
Age 74
Lakewood, WI

At the reunion of the High School Class of 1940, several hundred attended and of those who did not, many were disabled or deceased. How could this be? We were all about the same age, 72 or 73. The answers may be lost forever, but it is certain that some were the victims of smoking and other victims of heart attacks caused by over indulgence, some were the victims of excessive drinking. How smart we thought we were when in high school we engaged in those activities that were detrimental to our health. We were young and invincible and we could quit any time we want to. How wrong we were.

Those temptations are still present along with one we were never exposed to, drugs. Do you want to live to the age of your grandparents and still live an active, useful life? Or do you want to be disabled by an illness or disease that you could have prevented? The decision is yours and only you can make the choice. At the time of your 55th high school reunion will you be one of the healthy ones or just another name under "In Memory Of?"

Make your choice *now*.

WYOMING

Pearl Ashland
Age 72
Worland, WY

If you are going to live longer, enjoy the years as they go by. You are 20 years a child, 20 years a parent, another 20 as wage earner and mate. Then comes good times or bad depending on health and wealth.

Wealth does not depend on how much, but how you enjoy what you have. If it is a minimum amount, be selfish and spend it only on yourself. If you have lots of money, know the enjoyment of sharing with others. It may be family, friends, or institutions but give locally so you know where it goes and who it helps.

Health is a toss-up between what you feed the body and brain and the genes you have inherited. I believe the mind controls the body so what you enter into your computer each day is important. Enjoy your friends, ignore any slights or slurs. Don't be swallowed by family and laugh at every opportunity. Plus, just be moderate in everything that you enjoy, be it smoking, drinking, or eating. Why live to be 100 if it is no fun along the way!

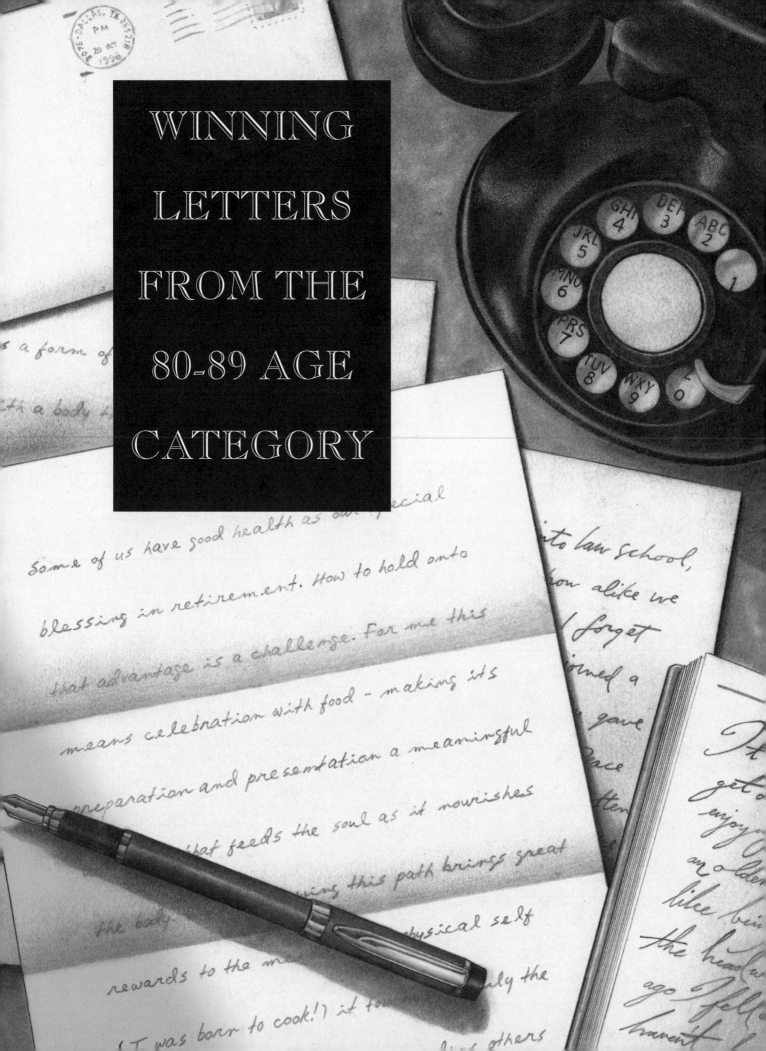

WINNING LETTERS FROM THE 80-89 AGE CATEGORY

Art Linkletter

A television and radio star for more than 60 years, ART LINKLETTER has performed in two of the longest running shows in broadcast history—*House Party*, which ran on daytime CBS-TV and radio for 25 years, and *People Are Funny* which ran on night-time NBC-TV and radio for 19 years. He has won two Emmy Awards and received four Emmy nominations; has received a Grammy Award; ten honorary doctorate degrees; and has also received other awards, honors, and recognitions too numerous to list. It should be noted that among those honors, is one in which he takes particular pride—Grandfather of the Year. *Kids Say the Darndest Things*—one of the top 14 best-sellers in American publishing history —and #1 for two consecutive years—is one of 23 books Art Linkletter has written. His most recent national best seller is *Old Age Is Not for Sissies*. Equally well known as a businessman, Art has served on many Boards of Directors including MGM, Western Airlines, Kaiser Hospitals, and the French Foundation for Alzheimer's Disease...to name but a few.

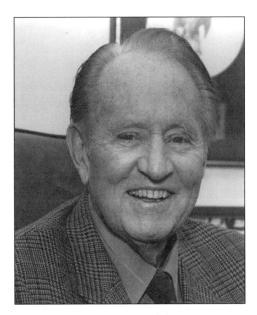

LONGEVITY

For the past 10 years I have been busy pursuing the subject of positive aging. Living better—longer—are the words that guide my studies in the field of positive aging. As president of the Center on Aging at UCLA, I meet with top scientists, philosophers, and social workers to explore the important subject of how to grow older and make the most of the later years. Therefore, I was delighted to be able to act as a judge in the Healthy Aging Letter-writing contest, and to see so many wonderful experiences described that fortify and enhance my own background of research into the subject. The variety of lifestyles and the even wider variety of advice given in these letters reinforces my determination to learn more and do better in this vital area.

By the year 2050, people over 65 will constitute more than one-fourth of our population and the revolutionary changes that will occur in our society as a result of this longevity will be startling and challenging. I am sure that as you read these winning letters you will be inspired with the down-to-earth practicality as well as the inspiring nature of their stories. No bureaucratic gobbledegook here! The words are from the heart and the advice is based on real life experiences that we can all learn from.

As an 85-year-old active senior, I salute my colleagues in this effort and find myself in my own life following most of their advice. Thus, I serve on a half dozen boards and run two or three businesses, lecture 50 to 60 times a year, write a book every three years, spend great vacation times with my eleven great-grandchildren, my nine grandchildren, my three children, and a wife with whom I have spent 61 years.

It's a great life!

ALABAMA

Arthur Forrester
Age 81
Lockhart, AL

I don't need a silly machine to keep my splendid and healthy body of 81 years—all I need to dismiss my sign of backache or stiffness is to lay on the floor for 15 or 20 minutes, first thing in the morning—like a cat after a nap I stretch in all directions. While lying there I think of faith, love, health, and contentment—these wonderful attributes attract the best environment.

Along with science I have proven false all the ideas and beliefs about old age, three score and ten length of life, the necessity of growing old and feeble.

Every so often on special occasions, I play a tape—music with a nice, easy going rhythm—I ad-lib a dance—then come happy feelings and my life a joyous adventure—devoid of stress.

ARIZONA

Frances Smith
Age 85
Nogales, AZ

Dear Future Generations of America:

I have discovered the most effective insurance for improving the physical, social, mental, or financial health of the aging is not something you can buy in a pharmacy. It is something you are already endowed with, and it's there to be used.

Now I know what my mother meant when she saw that I was depressed and said to me, "Think happy thoughts." Positive thinking will alleviate the stress of almost any worry, whereas dwelling on problems doesn't usually solve them but instead magnifies them, and you can actually worry yourself sick.

When you are stressed, mind over matter is a powerful tool. Try smelling the roses and enjoying a beautiful sunrise or sunset. Try doing a kind thing for somebody each day even if it is only a compliment, a friendly smile, or a pat on the shoulder.

Keep in mind the poet's advice, "Count that day lost whose low descending sun sets not upon some worthy action done."

And when you go to bed at night, give your troubles to God and you will not need a pill to sleep.

ARKANSAS

Ida Crane Walker
Age 87
Hot Springs, AR 71901

Rx For Healthy Living.

Dear Future Generations:

Have courage to do what you have to do. Accept life's adversities, recognize that which you can do nothing about, make the most of what you have, and share it.

Look outward. You'll see multitudes worse off than yourselves — physically, financially, and emotionally. Be grateful for your own good fortune.

When my infant was near death I asked my mother how she had gone on living after giving up one baby, much less four! She replied, "You do what you have to do."

In later years, faced with deaths of my youngest son and his four children when his plane exploded in mid-air, it would have been so easy to have joined them but my mother's advice, "You do what you have to do," saved me.

They're all gone now—parents, siblings, husband, my other two sons. I've been alone for 25 years, but never lonely. I'm still able to drive my car, can help others, am active in poetry and Toastmasters, and when night shadows fall, there's always a good book.

You, too, can have the good life.

From an octogenarian plus — who's been there.

CALIFORNIA

Albert L. Stern

Age 84

Diamond Bar, CA

Winston Churchill once said, "What we get makes a living . . . what we give makes a life." It is the retired person who can give, and perhaps make a life for someone else.

One lesson I learned was that while giving is of primary importance, enjoying the giving makes life really worthwhile. Life is stimulating when one looks forward to the challenge of helping others.

My youthful ambition was to become a lawyer. The depression of the 1930s prevented me from going to college, so I started working in a department store. Fifty years later I closed the variety store I had owned for 18 years. My wife and I had raised four children, all college graduates, and now I could retire.

On retirement I partially achieved my ambition by going to law school and becoming a paralegal. For the past 13 years I have been working and volunteering at Legal Services, which helps only those with very low incomes. I assist people with domestic violence problems with a case load of about 400 clients a year.

I know that my volunteer work helps others, not just myself, and most importantly I enjoy and look forward to each day.

COLORADO

Orien Johnson
Age 83
Colorado Springs, CO

Call me a talent scout. No, not for some sports team or beauty contest, but just to find talent in myself and in others.

I took a class in calligraphy and found out I had a talent for doing beautiful writing with a broad pen. I kept improving until I decided I was able to teach calligraphy to others. I went to a few senior centers, got permission to post some sign-up sheets, and started some classes.

At the first session I congratulate them for trying something new. "You don't want to be a couch potato, you want to keep learning. So do I." Then I say, "There's lots of talent in this room. It's been lying dormant inside of you. I'm going to find that talent, bring it out, polish it, and we'll see what happens."

So we take it a small step at a time, and I commend them for every bit of progress I see. It becomes a game, and everyone is a winner, including me.

Life-long learning is my goal. The more I learn and do, the happier I become. I'm shouting it from the housetops now: It's never too late!

CONNECTICUT

Lucia Eltgroth
Age 82
Trumbull, CT

There is nothing you can enjoy and nothing you can accomplish if you are sick. Therefore, first and foremost, take care of yourself.

You have been wonderfully made beyond anything man could do. But after functioning continuously for 70-80 years, parts begin to wear down. Attend quickly to those needing your intervention. Your body will do its own healing and cleaning if you don't overwhelm it with chemicals and medications. Be patient, it takes a little time to do that. You are advised to take your car for periodic check-ups if you want it to be reliable. Your body deserves at least that much consideration.

When you are well, your mind will be alert, your energy will remain high, your spirit will soar with joy, your heart will be able to love, and your age won't matter whatever it may be.

DELAWARE

Lillian Pearson
Age 80
Harrington, DE

To Whom it May Concern:

I was born in 1916. My parents tried to instill in me right from wrong. I didn't listen too well. Years of willfulness, hardship, and illness piled up.

When I surrendered my life and will to Jesus Christ, my life started to take on purpose and meaning. Then I was diagnosed with a deadly illness. God gave me a miracle of healing enabling me to return to work. I rose to the position of plant manager. This enabled me to live a healthy and comfortable retirement.

Other blessings were a good marriage, a daughter, a grandson, and a granddaughter. My grandchildren have six healthy sons and one lovely daughter. I also enjoy a host of good friends.

It is impossible to convey the joy and richness of my life in so few words. But knowing Christ in a personal way made the real change in my outlook on life.

Healthy Aging for me has been faith in and commitment to God, enabling me to realize my self-worth and value. Because God gives me peace and joy in myself, I can appreciate and reach out to others.

FLORIDA

Harvey E. Wagoner
Age 89
Sarasota, FL

The most important thing, after carefully selecting your grandparents, is moderation in all things.

Exercise is important. My dad did floor exercises in his nightshirts every morning. You should do ten minutes of floor calisthenics first thing every morning while you are still in your pajamas. Men should also use six pound dumbbells and women three pound ones. Walking is great exercise. I walk my nine-year-old Yorkiepoo dog every morning and evening.

Eat natural foods in moderation. The big meal should be at noon.

Marry someone in your 20s who is a good cook, a good nurse, has moral integrity, and intestinal fortitude.

Always spend one dollar less per month than what you earn.

When I was young, I played sandlot baseball. Later it was tennis, badminton, and finally golf. I fished all over Canada. I fished here in Sarasota, Florida from 1970-1980. Now my hobby for the last nine years is participating each week in a Life Story Writing Class.

After you are 65 years old do not move a refrigerator; do not climb up on the roof; and for heaven's sake, don't cross US41 at night wearing dark clothes.

GEORGIA

Eugenia V. Zellner
Age 80
Forsyth, GA

The day I became a grandmother 36 years ago, the aging process began in full force and almost overwhelmed me before I realized that I would have to find a new focus in my life, if I hoped to be my own person again.

What to do? Floundering, I enrolled in the graduate school of a nearby university, and by graduation day, I had found my calling—teaching social studies to high school and college level students, which I did until age 70.

Along with teaching, I did extensive traveling. Then I added modified aerobics three days a week and joined Weight Watchers to learn to eat more healthfully and to lose a few pounds.

A challenging vocation and an enjoyable hobby can do wonders for us mentally and physically. Growing and sharing roses is my oldest hobby. My newest hobby is writing notes to people who would appreciate one.

Every week I eagerly comb through our weekly newspaper to find names of people I know, of every age, who have won an honor, blocked a kick, celebrated an anniversary, or lost a loved one, and I write them a caring note.

This makes them happy and me healthy!

HAWAII

George Chaplin
Age 82
Honolulu, HI

A 16-year-old boy from Poland, dreams in his eyes, stood in awe as the ship passed the Statute of Liberty. Soon he would be in America, the land of freedom and opportunity.

He got a 12-hour-a-day job and went to night school to learn English. He persevered, and over time, he prospered. He was my father.

By example, during his 84 years, he shaped my philosophy of living and Healthy Aging:

* Wake each day to the joys of life—the sunshine, the bugle call of birds, the laughter of children, the smiles of flowers.

* Think young, for dreams need never retire.

* Respect your body and keep it fit through intelligent exercise, appropriate diet, and adequate rest.

* Substitute love and faith for anxiety and stress.

* Realize that life is crippled by hate and prejudice, but ennobled by tolerance, compassion, and respect for diversity.

* Measure life not by years, but by quality of deeds, making the world a kinder, gentler place for having the privilege of occupying it.

In sum, do what you know is right, with your feet on the ground, but your eyes lifted to the hills, helping to make tomorrow better than today.

IDAHO

Marjorie Wartchow
Age 82
Idaho Falls, ID

Healthy Living for the Aged.

Arriving at the age of 82 years old has been somewhat of a surprise, since I didn't have good health as a child, teenager, or adult. I'll give you two helpful ideas that have been beneficial to me. First is a positive attitude and second is a good sense of humor. Several doctors and friends have commented on my having these two attributes. Here is an example of what I mean. After a recent examination, my doctor asked me, "How are you feeling?" I answered him, "Well, as you know, I have reoccurring cancer, heart trouble, and high blood pressure, but I feel good!" Smiling, my doctor commented, "You say that you feel good?" "Yes, when I don't have an attack of Meniere's syndrome." By now he was laughing and asked again, "But you feel good?" I gave him the rest of my condition, "I'm legally blind, 70 percent of my hearing is gone, I'm losing my hair, and my teeth are falling out, but I feel good!" By the time I left, he was almost rolling on the floor! I think I made his day! So, that is my secret for healthy living. Attitude and humor! Faith and prayers won't hurt either! Try it, you'll like it!

ILLINOIS

Wycliffe McCracken
Age 89
Schaumburg, IL

Rx For a Healthy, Happy Life.

One opens the door to a healthy, enjoyable life via the perfect key, love—but do not use today's unfit key called love which seemingly requires immediate self-gratification. True love thinks of others' needs first and insists upon laughter, and humor that does not hurt one's fellow mortals.

I gave up nicotine and alcohol 89 years ago, at birth.

When marriage beckoned I hoped for an attractive wife with a strong sense of morality, coupled with an intoxicating humor . . . one who would enjoy our bed but would consider it relating to ourselves alone. I have been incredibly blessed with such a woman for 62 years.

These blessings, linked with calluses earned by hard labor contributed to health, a livable pension, and I hope, to community enrichment.

Though confined to a walker today, I manage essential exercise by household chores.

I follow the Hippocratic suggestion, "Let food be your medicine and medicine be your food."

Sleep remains a problem, for since I create and direct community theater, tomorrow's problems promise pleasurable excitement.

I have found that rather than counting sheep, it is better to talk to and *listen to* one's Shepherd.

INDIANA

Sr. Marien Plotzke
Age 83
Donaldson, IN

Dear Friends:

It's been a long time since I lived in a small home with my parents and brothers and sisters. We were always comfortable and never lacked what we needed even though we did not always have what we wanted. Our parents taught us how to enjoy simple things.

I remember one Christmas when my parents couldn't afford a new doll for me. As a surprise, Mom made a new outfit for my old doll and Dad made a cradle out of discarded pieces of wood. I never enjoyed a Christmas present as much!

Early in life I learned to enjoy simple things and to be satisfied with what I had and not thinking too much about what I would like. This proved valuable all through my life. It made me aware of all the beautiful things that are gifts of God and free: the lovely flowers of spring, the brilliant leaves as they change in fall, the songs of the birds, and the voices of faithful friends. None of these cost a cent and still they filled my life with beauty and enjoyment.

IOWA

G. Edgar Folk, Jr.
Age 82
Iowa City, IA

Dear Future Generations of America:

I am 82 years old and classified as Emeritus at a university. My family thinks I should be lying on a beach in Bermuda and reading novels. But I work full-time without pay at my career of physiologist because I enjoy my work so much. The happiest "retirees" I know are people who continue to set goals and pursue them with passion. If you can, choose work that inspires you with passion.

My other passions include horse shows and art gallery retrospectives, walking a mile a day, and dancing regularly to the big bands. The dancing keeps me in condition so I can travel on tour ships to Antarctica, where I deliver lectures on the polar environment and wildlife, then clamber into zodiac boats and over polar hills.

Another passion is the cabin I am building, where I plan to ski with friends this winter. If I work hard on the cabin, my reward is to walk through some delightful woods, looking for wild turkey, deer, badger, or wood duck, while picking up firewood delivered to the ground from the oak trees for my Franklin stove. Connecting with nature is crucial to well-being.

A variety of interests helps you stay healthy in mind, body, and soul. Invest in your passions; they repay handsomely in later life!

KANSAS

Wyeth W. Porr
Age 82
Pittsburg, KS

Dear Future Generations:

When you reach your senior years, you find yourself recalling your younger years. When you can find a caring ear, you gladly share the memories of your youth. You find yourself rambling on about your accomplishments and experiences—good and bad. You glorify your contributions to society. You magnify your importance in each act. You exaggerate your friendships. You flaunt the difference you have made. You remind the listener of the success you've harvested. You hungrily search for respect. You eagerly await the opportunity to give of yourself. You've learned that in the end all you have are your memories. You regret only the things you did not do. You think back to the times when you sat on the sidelines and watched *others* participate and reap the rewards. You now realize how important it is to take advantage of every opportunity that comes to you when you are young so that when you face your final years you will have true experiences, long-lasting friendships, and meaningful achievements to reminisce about with the younger generation. The young will not ignore you but eagerly anticipate their time with you and the wisdom you can offer them.

KENTUCKY

Dollie Galbraith
Age 83
Lexington, KY

If we had been asked years ago to describe our lives at 70 or 80 we would probably have used the words decrepit, dull, and uninteresting. However, as we enter these years, luckily, most of us are able to discredit these notions. Science and medicine have done much to enhance our lives, but never underestimate our determination to live life to its fullest. We should strive to keep our minds open to new ideas and not become cynical and opinionated. We are caretakers of our bodies and should do everything in our power to keep them healthy by diet, exercise, and positive thinking. To me, volunteerism has been the answer to healthy aging. It gives me an opportunity to enlarge my circle of friends, to become involved in community life and to intensify my feeling of self-worth. Most of all, volunteering gives me the chance to share my good fortune with those who are less fortunate.

LOUISIANA

Mrs. Marian Higgins
Age 88
New Orleans, LA

Next month I will be 89. When I turned the pages of each calendar during most of those years, I thought, "This is the best time of my life!"

As a child I greatly admired the character Pollyanna, the "Glad Girl," heroine of my favorite book. Pollyanna could always find something to be glad about in any situation. This matched my mother's slogan, "Everything happens for the best." I adopted that philosophy — and it has been a great help through the years. It helped me get through adolescence, the Great Depression, birth of three children, my husband's involvement in World War II, loss of my mother and later my husband, plus a long illness.

Another great aid to living is *empathy*. I didn't learn that word until I was in college. The dictionary says it means "the capacity of participating in another's feelings and ideas." Empathy has since been my guide in social life and business, but particularly in family life.

Over all this is *faith*. This great gift brings God close wherever you are. I acknowledge His help in following these guides through a long, happy life.

MAINE

Mrs. Robrita Brann
Age 81
Augusta, ME

When my husband retired at age 65 we did all the right things. We swam at the YMCA, attended exercise classes, and took lots of trips to see our country.

But the aging process inevitably caught up with us. The slowing step, the stiffening joint are not to be denied, and when illness and death caught up with my husband it left me in a vast state of nothingness. I needed a purpose, to feel useful again in some way.

Remembering how great the Health Reach Home Care nurses had been during my husband's illness, I contacted them, and eventually joined their Friendly Home Visitors program. Our job is to visit shut-ins.

A shut-in may be an elderly patient who just needs someone to talk to. It may be an accident victim confined while injuries are healing. It could be an expectant mother whose doctor has ordered bed rest in order to complete a difficult pregnancy.

So on two afternoons a week that is what I do. I have found if you brighten someone else's day, it will surely brighten yours. The secret to Healthy Aging? Smile — and keep moving. It's as simple as that.

MARYLAND

Marian B. See
Age 80
Baltimore, MD

How do I turn autumn years from gray to golden? I volunteer.

Volunteering satisfies my need to remain useful at my own pace, and in life's mainstream instead of on the sidelines.

Volunteering challenges me to maintain healthy habits, knowing someone depends on my continued fitness.

Volunteering exercises my mind and spirit, as well as these arthritic bones, to keep me flexible and unafraid of change.

Volunteering permits payback for the education I was privileged to receive, the skills I was able to acquire, when I contribute time and energy to worthwhile causes.

Volunteering encourages me to look for hidden talents and resources in those I work with.

Volunteering allows me to give graciously, whatever my financial situation.

Yes, I'm preparing for the season's gusty winds, but determined to resist the blight of frost and paint my bit of color across life's landscape.

MASSACHUSETTS

Ethelind E. Austin
Age 87
Norton, MA

Dear Friends:

Keeping active is the one single thing
That gives my life its zip and zing.

At age 87 I still ride my bicycle,
(At age 97 I'll downsize to a tricycle!).

They say of me, "She enjoys
Whatever cuts down on avoirdupois."

So, join me, don't just empathize
with my aerobic exercise.

I do my share of volunteering
(Ignoring being hard of hearing.)

Puzzles and word games keep me jumping;
Hefting Webster's and Bartlett's keeps me pumping.

I write many letters, at least one a week,
To absent friends, both young and antique.

"Neither snow, nor rain, . . . nor gloom of night"
Delays my letters on their flight.

To wherever I wish, inland or coastal,
Thanks to the U.S. Service Postal!

I go to the P.O. seeking replies;
I might win a contest — what a surprise!

So, for octogenarians, this thought I impart —
Let's all be active, and young at heart.

MICHIGAN

Florence L. Lampshire
Age 82
Flint, MI

There are many rules for being happy and healthy as we travel toward the latter part of our life's journey. Each one has its merits and should have our attention.

The one I would give the highest priority is that of keeping in touch with other people, entering into their lives, and taking them into our own. Family relationships are the most valuable, but for complete fulfillment we need to reach beyond the family circle and become involved with others.

For me, this has been accomplished through joining a penpal group, and I correspond with more than a hundred pen friends around the world. It is rare when a single day's mail brings less than six letters, and sometimes there are a dozen or more.

We help each other through painful experiences, and we rejoice together over the happy occasions. People are the same the world over, though the addresses vary. For nine years, my mailbox has contained letters from West Malaysia, France, Germany, Brazil, Africa, Scotland, Australia, and England, along with many from the United States and Canada.

We are all members of a very special family, sharing joys and sorrows, always knowing we are not alone.

MINNESOTA

Elsie Solberg
Age 84
Buffalo, MN

Dear Tommy:

Are you ready for your journey through life? I've been on that fascinating trip for 84 years, and I've become an expert packer. Here—let me help you with your backpack. Take these things from my heart and hands and gently pack them:

Faith: Have faith in your creator and in yourself. You are special. No one on earth is exactly like you.

Hope: Hope that you will find the elusive quality that makes you who you are and who you will become.

Peace: Be peaceful; practice a stillness of spirit that comes from touching other lives to make them better.

Love: Give unconditional love that makes everyone you meet your friend. Give love and receive it abundantly.

These companions—Faith, Hope, Peace, and Love—will bring you the good things in life: joy and sadness; laughter and tears; humility and compassion; tolerance and understanding; fulfillment and happiness.

Oftentimes we travel with too much baggage. If your backpack becomes too heavy, discard it, but always keep unconditional love. It will protect and sustain you as you walk onward to make life your dreams or your dreams your life.

I wish you Godspeed, my young friend!

MISSISSIPPI

Frances Antley
Age 89
Forest, MS

Dear Adult Friend:

If a mean mother made you eat turnip greens
And much other nutritional food
Love was what made her do it
She knew it was for your own good.

First, she gave you milk and watched you grow
Then, *I will give good juices* she would think.
No alcohol would ever be in her plan
For her precious child to drink.

If she caught you smoking a cigarette
The danger to your lungs she would declare
Telling you of cancer and other bad diseases
And warning you of polluting others' air.

She encouraged you to play lots of games
She knew exercise was good for you.
The social aspect of making good friends
Was a plus in your character too.

If you listened to mother and took her advice
You should be a healthy adult by now.
Whether fifty or seventy or far beyond
Her ways were best, you will proudly vow.

The main ingredients for a happy family life
Are Love, Faith, and Trust in everyone
With these traits and sensible health rules
Why not live to be a hundred and one?

MISSOURI

Ralph O. Fritts
Age 89
Amsterdam, MO

Write a letter to inspire future generations about healthy aging — physically, socially, mentally, or financially? A challenge, but I'll try.

What qualifications do I have? The first would be my good health, physically and mentally, at age 89. Socially, all that involves a lifetime of schooling, business, social and military service, and family. Last, a financial standard that should be adequate.

As the youngest of 15 children, I was reared in a home where laughter was a way of life, and hard times were only an inconvenience. The government existed only to govern and one's well-being was a personal problem. In practice rather than words my parents managed to convey to their large brood a belief in self-reliance that would serve them well in later years. That reliance must be cultivated if our nation is to remain strong.

Develop an acceptance of the problems of life, for they are *your* problems. This fact was expressed so well by a former president in his oft-quoted desk sign, "The Buck Stops Here."

MONTANA

Elsie Kolashinski
Age 84
Great Falls, MT

To live a fuller life, concentrate on the present to keep your mind alert and healthy. This awareness helps create memories that will increase in value with age. Visit the past but don't live there. Have hopes and dreams. Look ahead anticipating good, but don't escape into a dream world. Memories and dreams are important, but *learn to live in the now*!

Pause and listen to a bird's song. Try to identify the bird. Examine leaves and flowers, including weeds. Really see them, marvel at their individual beauty. Smell the flowers, notice that trees, rain, even dust have distinctive odors. The smallest stone holds a story from centuries past. Become aware of their varied beauty. Learn more about them. When you bite into an apple or crisp stalk of celery, feel the little bursts of flavor. Enjoy the feel and smell of food as well as the taste.

If, due to increasing age or other cause, you are deprived of any of your senses or abilities, concentrate on and intensify the use of others. Increased awareness brings new knowledge. Share it. Learn to listen. In every way become aware of *now* and savor each moment.

NEBRASKA

Ruth Boellstorff
Age 87
Brock, NE

Dear Fellow Traveler:

Long experience on life's road has convinced me that happy Healthy Aging can best be achieved by developing positive social attitudes. To that end I offer here some tried-and-true rules for those who follow me.

Smile a lot; it hides the wrinkles.

Be careful with criticism. It's a two-edged sword.

Resist the temptation to recount your aches and pains.

Marvel over new things. Learn something new at every opportunity.

Don't feel you must express an opinion on every subject.

Remind yourself there are few things more unpleasant than a sour complaining old person.

Exercise! If you can't run, walk. If you can't walk, push that wheelchair to the limit.

Refrain from sharing your vast experience. Unsolicited advice is never welcome.

Never relax your standards of personal grooming. "Age which forgives itself is forgiven nothing." (G.B.Shaw)

Find something in everyone to sincerely admire.

Praise the efforts of others.

Praise others.

Praise God.

NEVADA

Jack F. Moore
Age 82
Las Vegas, NV

I'm a 1914 model, in my eighth decade. Each decade was interesting, fascinating, different, and at times, difficult. During difficult times my dad would quietly say, "Everything in moderation." He recommended moderation in such things as eating, drinking, driving. Good advice.

Before 1960 we knew little about diet, vitamins, workouts. Then came the fitness explosion!

Diet. My generation ate three meals a day, breakfast, ham and eggs; lunch and dinner, meat, potatoes, gravy, desserts. Today, in our home, we eat one main meal daily, at midday. This usually consists of salad, fresh fruits and vegetables, fish or chicken, light dessert. Breakfast, fruit or juice, whole wheat toast or cereal. Light snack in evening if desired. Drink eight glasses of water daily, even if not thirsty.

Vitamins. My doctor said, "Unnecessary. Just eat a balanced diet." Balanced diet? Every day? We began taking vitamins. Today my doctor takes (and recommends) vitamins. Vitamins, it seems some doctors were the last to know.

Workouts. Health club membership fine but not necessary. What is important is daily exercise, such as walking, swimming, cycling, always include stretching exercises. Make it a daily habit. "Just do it."

Finally, remember my dad? "Everything in moderation."

NEW HAMPSHIRE

Florence Byrd Woods
Age 87
Bath, NH

Dear Class of 2000 A.D.:

A cistern is a tank that gets its water from a never-failing spring up on a hillside. The water is piped into the cistern and can leave by an overflow pipe, so it is always cold, clean, and clear.

You can take a dipper to drink from the cistern whenever you are thirsty.

My recipe for Healthy Aging is simple:

Drink from your own cistern.

This is of course a metaphor, but metaphors are true. You do have such a wellspring deep within yourself. Once you find it, and you can, you can take your dipper and drink. If you do this freely and often, you will find your own true bent and the path you must follow. You will begin to love the person you were meant to be; you will love other persons, and you will find joy and humor in life itself, come what may. For the spring up on the hillside is never-failing. Its waters are health to your whole being.

Bon Voyage!

NEW JERSEY

Mary Annicelli
Age 83
Toms River, NJ

Dear Aging Americans:

It's human to regret the passing of youth — the loss of virility and agility. Mourn not that loss. Remember, those years carried many heavy burdens. Divest yourself of those shackles of the young. Youth is over. Don't look back in sorrow or longing. If you carried your burdens well, you can now rest on your laurels. If your past wasn't all you had hoped for or planned, nothing you can do will change it.

So, gather up the sadness, failures and disappointments. Bury them, bury them in the deepest recesses of your mind.

Now forward! Be free! As you approach the sunset years, each day can be a building block to a fine life. You don't have to search for happiness. It's all around you. Seek it in your own heart. Rise each morning and know that the day is a new beginning. If you give full measure of devotion to living, you are a success. Past lessons learned have made you strong.

In the final analysis, I believe a good attitude contributes to good health and good health engenders a good attitude. Life can be full and rewarding.

You can make your own utopia.

NEW MEXICO

William A. Diven
Age 82
Las Cruces, NM

Dear Lads and Lassies:

In a nation obsessed with the idea of remaining young at all cost, you may have difficulty believing that the aging process can be a most unforgettably rewarding and joyous experience, but let me assure you that such is true.

This can never be a reality, however, unless you are willing, as you traverse life's highways and pot-holed roads, to put forth serious efforts to accomplish such a goal. It does not just happen.

Oh, I could offer you a definitive guide detailing various steps to be followed in order to reach that goal, but, after much, much thought, I have concluded that only one recommendation deserves the most serious consideration of all.

Unless you are willing and able to rid yourself of all the personal, emotional garbage (hate, fear, envy, jealousy, hurt, self-centeredness, and the like) that can accumulate like barnacles on a ship, and smother your heart, soul, and mind, you will never be free to experience life as a memorable adventure, and retirement as a golden opportunity to enjoy life to its fullest.

The choice is yours.

NEW YORK

Simeon Baron
Age 86
Yorktown Heights, NY

Snow on the Roof.

As the old adage states, "There may be snow on the roof, but down in the basement furnace the embers glow merrily."

If you had told me in my youth that love, romance, and sexual attraction was still vibrant in a 60 to 90 age group, I would have laughed with a smirk plus a raised wiggling of the eyebrows.

True, the emotion of love at my senior condominium village is at a slower, placid pace, but it is there! The smiles, the pleasantries, the liaisons are all positives in this life-pursuit of health and happiness.

Good old Philadelphian Benjamin Franklin continually wrote about the advantages of courting an older woman.

My feelings are always reverent when I see an older couple strolling down the lane, holding hands.

Down in balmy Florida, the Rip Van Winkles and the Barbara Frietchies have coupled in the thousands, they all refer to each other as, "My Boy Friend" or "My Girl Friend." Most of these romances lean to the mental attitude, yet there are a few vestiges of physical activity.

So, for health, happiness, and well-being at any age latch on the *ye olde tyme romance*.

Toujours L'Amour

NORTH CAROLINA

Harriet L. Hayne
Age 88
Chapel Hill, NC

On Being a Grandmother.

As I age, I have been surprised to discover how much being a grandmother means to me. It has contributed not only to the day-to-day pleasures of my life but also to my general well-being.

I take pride in my grandchildren's achievements (they are now proceeding through their 20s) and in the warm affection that marks our exchanges. They keep me alert as their birthdays chart the months and days of the year. But more seriously, as I read the daily news, I clip and send them accounts close to their interest: to Ted the Third World volunteer, news of floods in Bangladesh; to Alison, the budding naturalist, news of an internship to study wolves. Then, would a check to Margaret help pay for that special course? And perhaps Terry would like another paperback from my collection of mysteries.

Lastly, to be there when they may need me, I try to keep up my strength (why else would I go to the pool so faithfully?) and ponder how best to preserve my worldly assets.

At this moment in my life, being a grandmother provides me a road, royal indeed, to Healthy Aging.

NORTH DAKOTA

Marguerite H. Hubbard
Age 80
Fargo, ND

Learn to understand and like yourself. You are the one person you must live with all of your life. One's talents are not equal. Natural talents manifest themselves, but must be developed. Recognize and analyze your physical and/or mental limitations.

If possible strengthen your weak areas. If they are not subject to change just accept them and build on your strengths. Your particular strengths may be physical, social, intellectual, thoughtful, analytical, loyal, and combinations of these and other traits.

Recognize opportunities available to you. Be willing to accept direction and advice. Actively seek both from persons you admire, and know have your best interests at heart. They may be relatives, teachers, neighbors, friends, or employers. Many might not offer advice, but are willing to share their observations if asked.

We are not all destined to be rocket scientists, beauty queens, or star athletes. The world needs competent truck-drivers and mechanics, caring nurses, cheerful friendly sales and service personnel, child and elder care attendants. All make life better and easier for others.

Accept yourself. Be content. Happiness is internal. Contentment is a personal achievement. Find your niche. Do your best, and angels can't do better.

OHIO

Dorothy L. Hershey
Age 88
Dayton, OH

Age is a matter of the mind and if you don't mind it doesn't matter.

In 1979, I retired at the age of 71 after having spent 50 years in retail. I knew that I would never be happy in that rocking chair. So my husband and I joined the ranks of the Retired Senior Volunteer Program. We found a great deal of satisfaction in our volunteer years, doing something for someone else. One meets a lot of nice people and it keeps that brain matter alert. We worked for many agencies, Red Cross, Cancer Society, the United Way, the Dayton Foundation, Children's Services to name a few. Along the way we formed a group of six women who have worked together on many projects. I lost Mr. Hershey four years ago but have continued with the group that he headed. When one gets up in the morning and has something to do one doesn't have time to get bored. Volunteerism is my answer to Healthy Aging—don't know what I would do without it.

I am now approaching my 89th year, on the go by public transportation three to four days a week—grateful to be able to do it.

OKLAHOMA

Josephine H. Spivey
Age 80
Oklahoma City, OK

Dare!

As a teen, I was inspired by a little book called "I Dare You." I dared!

The dare? Be square, to be well-rounded.

Physical

Social ☐ Mental ◯

Spiritual

Balance the physical, intellectual, spiritual, and social to make a well-rounded person.

Health is primary. So I exercise, eat right, think positively, do not abuse with alcohol, drugs, cigarettes, or anger.

Then what about the spiritual me? Essential to an inner peace, for me, I must read my Bible, pray, attend church, tithe, and be kind to others.

Which comes to a social me. Friendship needs cultivating. So I try to lend a helping hand, offer encouragement, give a smile—sometimes a hug.

Yet who will enjoy my company if I am a dullard? Mental growth must not be neglected. I received a law degree and journalism degree while holding a full-time job. Yet there is so much to learn. Am I too old to tackle the Internet and world wide web? Even Jesus "increased in wisdom and stature, and in favor with God and man." (Luke 2:52)

So at age 80, I must keep trying *to do the best I can, with what I have, wherever I am*. Join me.

OREGON

John M. Poorman
Age 85
Portland, OR

Recently I saw an old dog walking alone along a downtown sidewalk. My first thought was that the dog would be killed by the heavy traffic at the next intersection. My second thought was he didn't get to be an old dog by being stupid. Worry not. He stopped at the intersection and waited for people to cross and he simply crossed with them.

We too may no longer be as nimble as we were when younger, but we do know how to compensate. Without discounting good genes, somewhere along the way those of us over 85 must have done something right. Age does not necessarily make us wise, but to be a survivor, certain insights must somehow have been assimilated. Perhaps we won without consciously trying.

We have learned to laugh, eat right, exercise within limits, and keep our brains in gear. Everyone has trials and tribulations from time to time so maybe the key is how we cope come good times and bad. So who's old? Who's mature? Except for getting a discount if over 65, what differentiates us from the kids? (Everyone younger than I am is a kid.)

Frankly, I love these elegant years.

PENNSYLVANIA

Amy L. McIntyre
Age 85
Tionesta, PA

I have no inspiring words to impart. Only that life is wonderful. What we make of it is up to us. We can let tragedy make us turn bitter, or make us grow. God is always there to help us bear our load, and He gives us grace to carry our share.

The darkest hour is before dawn. Dawn always comes, giving a new day, and new hope.

Humor is also important. If you can find a speck of humor in a problem, it is already half solved.

I note that in a long weary line at a checkout, when my eyes meet another weary one, if I smile, their face lights up, and the shoulders lift, and I feel good.

I do not sit back and wait for others to do for me. If my body can't, my mind will, and if it doesn't, my lips do.

I am on a very tight budget, but I find enjoyment in marking "paid" behind each item at the end of the month, and if there is a dollar over, it's a lovely bonus.

Life is indeed wonderful!

RHODE ISLAND

Camella Zampini
Age 81
Hope Valley, RI

Hi Everyone!

I am 81 years young. I don't feel old yet or act my age. I enjoy kidding and joking because laughter is the best medicine I find. It works for me. I'm careful about what foods I choose to eat. I enjoy lots of fruits and veggies. No fatty food! No liquor, soda, or drugs. I drink eight glasses of water daily and take long walks each day. Smile even though you're crying on the inside.

It does a body good. Try to be kind and considerate to someone. It works wonders. Does your heart good too. I enjoy writing poetry about people who do their utmost for others and to say thanks. I now have six scrapbooks full of letters and cards from people in all walks of life. I live on a small income but I'm careful how I spend it. I also took care of my dad who was crippled and confined to a wheelchair for five heartbreaking years until he died. I took care of my brother who died of lung cancer. Because I care, the good Lord has rewarded me in more ways than one. I'm still here. Thanks Lord.

SOUTH CAROLINA

William A. Reeves
Age 87
Summerville, SC

During the Great Depression I adopted a philosophy that has served me well. I attribute much of my mental, physical, social, and financial well-being to it.

As a New Yorker I have a proclivity for catch phrases. In my graduation book a classmate gave me credit for "don't never ever worry." This was in 1927, and we couldn't imagine what the future would bring.

But in the dark days that soon came I found that "*Don't worry about those things over which you have no control*" kept me reasonably sane.

This doesn't mean a lack of concern about you or your family, for that would be avoiding the responsibility that is a part of maturity. It means your concern must be coupled with action taken to resolve the problem. Don't waste energy in useless worry.

When events occur that seem at first impossible to resolve, take an action! If it appears unsuccessful it helps to clear your mind, and eventually to result in a successful conclusion.

Now at 87, with several ailments, I can still anticipate each day and uncounted blessings surround me.

SOUTH DAKOTA

Shirley Baughman O'Leary
Age 82
Belle Fourche, SD

Dear Person of the Future:

To help you toward a healthy old age, my experience suggests that you should keep an open heart to all of God's creation: Be interested, be observant, be concerned, be appreciative.

Enjoy nature: Get out and walk in it, observe its birds, animals and plants, its rocks and waters, its scenic vistas — and work to preserve them for others.

Be interested in people of all kinds and try to help those who need help. Value especially your extended family, your link to the past and your comfort in the present, and a life partner who shares your goals.

Take good care of your health when you are young.

Try to find work which interests you, contributes something to the world, and brings you an income from which you can set aside money for a comfortable old age.

Have hobbies — reading, music, crafts, sports, and pets — which will enlarge your horizons and take you out of yourself.

Appreciate! Count your blessings and be thankful. Being part of a religious group will keep you mindful of them.

You can't close your mind to the bad things that happen, but keep looking for the good.

TENNESSEE

Richard R. Lewis
Age 89
Knoxville, TN

In July 1972, I reached 65, then the age for compulsory retirement. That ended 43 years of steady work. I tried to tell myself termination didn't matter, but actually I was despondent and spent my time watching TV and feeling useless. Being in good health, I didn't realize I was neglecting it.

Realization came in the fall of the next year, when I went to a Tennessee football game. I missed the kick-off because, on the stadium ramp, I huffed and puffed and had to rest.

Then it dawned on me, I had been following the path of least resistance, which went nowhere.

Next day, I called the boy who'd promised to rake my leaves and told him I'd do it myself. That was the beginning of my rejuvenation. Next, and of most help, I started a program of regular exercise at the "Y." Then after resuming contact with old friends, I found myself looking for something worthwhile to do in my spare time. That led to an interesting hobby, compiling a family history, including my memoirs, and giving copies to my children and close relatives. Other worthwhile activities followed, and I began to feel useful once more!

TEXAS

Faye Field
Age 84
Longview, TX

If I had known being old would be this great, I would not have stayed young so long.

Aging is a joy mentally.

I relish the time I now have for inspirational reading, in-depth research, and thorough rather than cursory examination of printed matter in my fields of interest.

I appreciate the growth of the mature mind which acquires an added tolerance in contrast to the judgmental attitude of earlier years.

I enjoy the challenge of letting my mind gain from past experiences which make the present comprehensible and the future beckoning.

Each day I read something uplifting, informative, or entertaining.

Aging brings about greater selectivity. Now I engage largely in only the best, whereas I formerly was satisfied with what I considered good or even fair.

I keep a daily journal which helps sharpen my powers of observation and intensifies my sensitivity to the exciting happenings around me.

I make an effort to appear alert, vibrant, and cheerful so that my younger friends will see that aging does not have to be synonymous with decline.

Lastly, I have come to believe that if we live long enough with open-mindedness and good will, we can understand everybody!

UTAH

Hazel Johns
Age 85
Orem, UT

Healthy Aging is an interesting and educational process. This journey through life, being filled with many exciting experiences, some wonderful and some not so great, makes life an exciting journey. As we go along we learn from our mistakes and each day we have the opportunity to improve our lives and do better.

Live each day as it comes along. To live in the past is not productive — to prepare for the future is wise — but to enjoy each day as it comes along makes life worth living — enjoy each moment.

If life brings hardships and discouragement remember—this too will pass—be optimistic.

One way to be happy is to go out and make someone else happy. It's not difficult to find someone who needs a friend or a helping hand. Opportunities are all around us — to do a service for someone or just "be there" for them makes this world a brighter and happier place.

Don't sit around and wait for it to be a good day — go out and make it a good day.

VERMONT

Catherine Wood
Age 83
Lyndonville, VT

Dear Friends:

It is great to write about a subject about which I have given much thought. I believe it is very basic for us to reverence our bodies by right foods; no abuses and the best of care. Each stage in life needs to be preparing us for the next, that we may be able to fulfill the purposes for which we have been put on this earth. Because I am aging, I do not believe I am necessarily getting old. Thus, I am able to keep learning and keep serving at 83 years of age.

It brings on the wrinkles when we give in to worry, doubt, fear, distrust, and despair. We are as young as our faith, as old as our doubt, as young as our enthusiasm, and as old as our fear, as young as our hope and as old as our despair.

I believe that with beauty, hope, cheer, courage, and grandeur generating our days in the presence of the Almighty, we will remain young and have Healthy Aging.

VIRGINIA

Robert R. Graham
Age 83
Hampton, VA

When I was young (high school and college) I wanted to learn to smoke. I tried, but inhaling the smoke made me dizzy and not inhaling it burned my tongue. At about 25 I decided it was foolish to try to learn to like something so distasteful. I made one of my life's wisest decisions.

At 27 I met the girl of my dreams. She took me home to meet her family and I met her 6´4˝ tall brother. I visualized being married to her and having a tall son like him. He had one failing: He smoked cigarettes.

I married my dream girl and after two daughters and 20 years of marriage, we had a son who grew tall and handsome like his uncle. However, he followed his father's example and at 33 he doesn't smoke. He is a successful Vice President at Lehman Brothers on Wall Street (and looking for his dream girl).

His uncle continued smoking even after having a diseased lung removed. He died at age 76 after several years' suffering.

I am now 83 and still going strong. How much longer could my brother-in-law have lived if he hadn't smoked?

WASHINGTON

LaRue Williams
Age 89
Enumclaw, WA

It is incredible that I, who had to take "Bone Head" English in college before I could enter Freshman English 1A, would enter a letter writing contest. I decided that it was my one big chance to tell the seniors that there is "Life After Moving." Moving brought on by one's children who insist that one should live near their offspring in later life. Even though these children carry post graduate degrees parents say, "What do they know?" Eventually the move is made.

Now is the time to repair the mental damage done by leaving the family home and the long time friends. Get Thee to the nearest Senior Center, church social, or "Bring Your Own Sandwich Group." Just remember they have been through the same stages of life as you.

They felt the sting of poverty during the Depression, carried their load during World Wars, were PTA presidents, and refereed Little League Games.

Canes, walkers, and wheelchairs do not keep one from playing cards or making warm friendships over lunch. You'll find it most rewarding to be with people who have met life "Head On!"

WEST VIRGINIA

Ruth Schwartz
Age 80
Charleston, WV

Dear Unknown Friends:

I enjoy writing for it keeps me mentally alert. When my thoughts transfer to paper, I am never alone.

Over the past 40 years, I have written to a girlhood friend. At first she had little to impart. Perhaps she enjoyed reading the way I expressed myself. Certainly she felt the warmth of my words.

Then I located a cousin on my mother's side of the family. Sanda and family lived in Romania. The family emigrated to Israel. Sanda said her English was "not good." I replied that by writing to me, it would improve. I wanted to greet her as family. My warmth reached her. Fifteen years have passed. Our letters are visual and consistent.

My love for writing has enlarged. I write poetry and short stories. I found my niche in children's stories. My imagination then knew no bounds for I became as one with my fictional characters. My grandsons were very pleased to read them. I have not been published.

Lord Byron aptly expressed himself: "Letter-writing is the only device of combining solitude with good company."

In my writing diversity, I humbly agree.

WISCONSIN

Virginia Dymond
Age 85
Madison, WI

Dear Prospector:

As I have grown older, I have now and then felt myself to be on a plateau where I can look back and view the paths and turns my life has taken. I see more than failures, successes, trauma, wounding, and shrinking income with more budgeting for medications. And though I have severe attacks of poverty, I am relived when they have passed, for the plateaus have also allowed a look at what I was and what I am.

The plateau experience has underlined and redefined my needs. The importance of stimulation and excitement from learning is alive and well, and love of books is strong. I need to continue to participate in life, but I am also an observer, and I note that growing elderly has given me a kind of freedom in being myself. I don't need to keep proving myself. What a plus! The importance of some things which once seemed clearly important has dimmed, but honesty and civility matter. Concentrate on enrichment of life. Books and art make a difference.

Life may be hard, but the plateaus show kindnesses and sometimes good luck, and I am grateful.

Best wishes

WYOMING

Betty L. Evenson
Age 86
Casper, WY

I am 86 years old and in possession of many of the ills that old people fall heir to. I'd like to give this bit of advice to those who will follow me.

Don't let it get you down. Don't lose your sense of humor.

Depression will come. We can't ignore the fact that there will be times of discouragement and frustration and rebellion. And let them come—you're entitled. Don't try to be a 24 hour a day hero.

There will a patch of bright blue shining beyond the falling leaves and something to smile about; the smell of pot roast coming from the kitchen at supper time, the touch of a caring hand smoothing the bedtime quilt around your shoulders.

Appreciate the little things. We had our good years and are thankful for them.

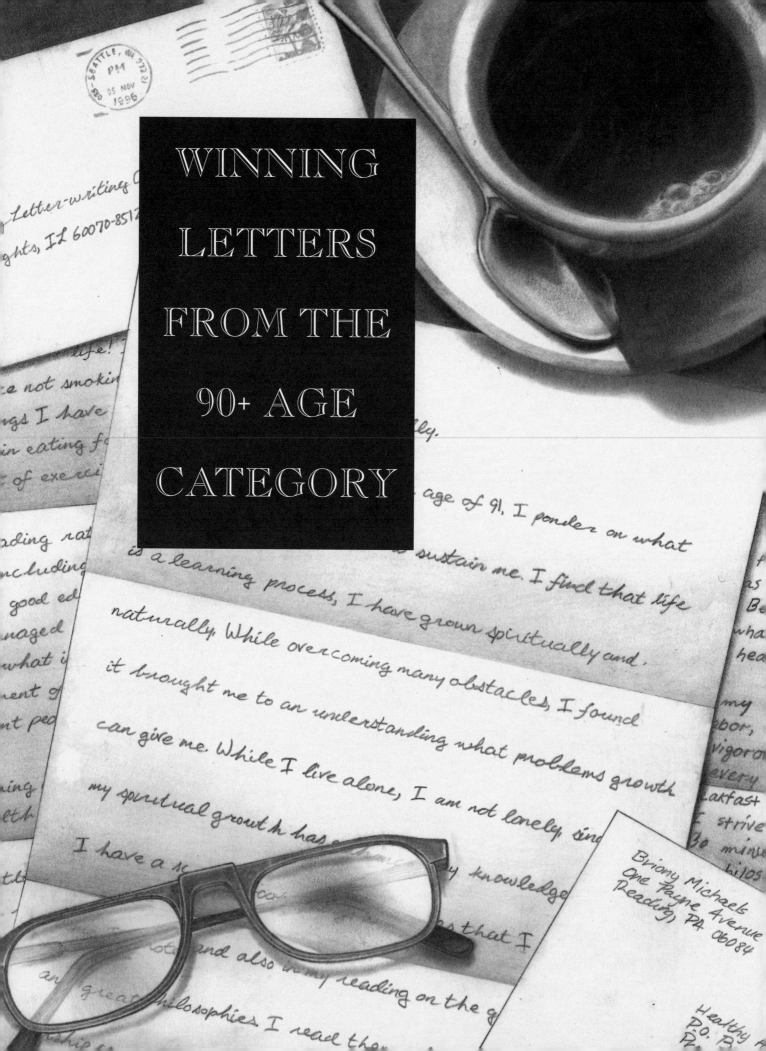

WINNING LETTERS FROM THE 90+ AGE CATEGORY

Ida Davidoff

IDA FISHER DAVIDOFF, Ed.D. is a 93-year-old marital and family therapist whose goal is to change attitudes about aging. A graduate of Simmons College with a masters from Radcliffe, she obtained a doctorate at age 58 from Columbia University Teachers College and has been in private practice for 43 years. Dr. Davidoff has published numerous professional papers and is a frequent inspirational lecturer on age-related topics, most of which are based on personal experience—what she's had to cope with during the aging process, and her clinical and theoretical synthesis of the solutions. Dr. Davidoff has been featured by ABC News with Diane Sawyer, and was profiled in two nationally aired public television specials: *Our Nation's Health... Healthy Aging and Healthy Aging ... Redefining America*. Her book in progress, which includes her "Decalogue on Aging," is titled *Youth: A Gift of Nature; Age: A Work of Art*. An expressed goal of Dr. Davidoff's has been "Down with Ageism."

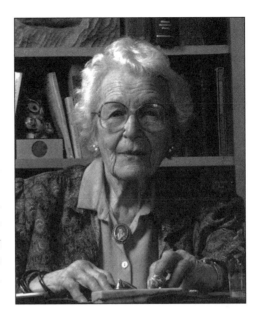

DOWN WITH AGEISM!

Today many of us live into the 80s, 90s and even 100s. It is imperative that with society's help and the individual's effort we live as vibrantly as possible, good mental and physical health be maintained. No two people are alike, nor does only one item determine Healthy Aging. In the past with religion a primary value, heaven was the goal. Today a long, healthy life has taken its place, from heaven to health.

It has been stated that aging is inevitable, that society imposes stereotypes and false negative expectations on us, but we can nevertheless create a unique vital self by following certain basics. This group of elders, 90 to 105 years old in their letters, have done just that. They are grateful for the gift of life, believe in God, treat their bodies with respect, "do not pour on alcohol, drugs, or smoke or even medical drugs," exercise daily, especially walking, eat fresh fruits, vegetables, grains, all in moderation, and have done so from childhood. (One exception of a never-missed breakfast of bacon, two eggs, buttered toast, and coffee!) They try to care for others as for the self, "when feeling lonely, it helps to make the effort to help someone else." Avoid debts, "you then are a slave to your debtor." There was little discussion of finances other than pride in independence. They fought obstacles, seeing them as a challenge and themselves not as victims.

Recent research on centenarians found similar trends, optimism, involvement in some aspect of life, relationships, ability to cope with change.

There was a pride in a "good memory" and respect for the kingdom of the mind. Lack of sharpness of the mind spelled deterioration of the body. Surprisingly no one referred to TV or the movies as a source of stimulation, but there were many references to reading, music, dancing, writing, volunteering, church activities, grandchildren, family, friends.

While we "oldsters" began life relying on our legs for reaching a destination, to school, church, a friend's house, library, or work, by cooking on a coal stove, by gas light, doing mental arithmetic in a world of limited horizons and limited aspirations, we have been resilient enough to fit comfortably into a world of airplanes, microwave ovens, computers, and limitless horizons. Education was less important when we were young. Very few went to college, most had some years of elementary school, but high school was only beginning to beckon.

The first and basic step in my own decalogue for Healthy Aging is coming to terms with the changes or "mourning-liberation," not as helpless, immobilized victims of the "impossibility of possibility," but freely creative fighters with endless curiosity and a zest for overcoming stereotypes, for avoiding unnecessary dependencies appropriately, keeping up with facts and new realities about aging, being needed, creating our own image and growing. On my banner is the slogan, "We do not grow old; we become old by not growing. Down with ageism."

ALABAMA

Anna Mary Harbin
Age 90
Montgomery, AL

Moderation.

Begin with morning prayer, learn to have hope, understanding and love for mankind, respect the good earth that nourishes you with the fruits it brings forth, and keep your allegiance to our beautiful U.S.A.

Be happy and laugh often, be not afraid and never give up!

I have lived the above from an early age and by the grace of God have reached this age healthy and peacefully.

There is a beauty about old age, my husband and I fought the world through joy and sorrow for 65 years, until he was taken by death.

We lived to enjoy our four children educated and married who gave us twelve grandchildren. What more could we ask for? You can too!

ALASKA

John L. Dolenc
Age 92
Palmer, AK

Having celebrated my 92nd birthday in April 1996 I was asked what I attributed my longevity to and my response then was *activity*. I always have a project ongoing and at least one for the future.

Activity includes plenty of hard physical work, exploring and pursuing new ideas, and being of active service to my community. I have served on various boards, search and rescue missions, committees, City Council, and Borough Assembly. I still take an active part in many Lions Club projects, the Masonic Lodge, and am currently serving on the Cemetery Board.

I consider it important to take good care of my health by eating nutritious foods. I do not use tobacco products. As important is keeping mentally alert by reading, studying financial reports, keeping up with current events, and getting proper rest. It is important to keep both a healthy mind and body.

For relaxation I enjoy the outdoors and have both fished and hunted in Alaska during the 60-plus years of living in this delightfully enchanting state.

ARKANSAS

Trudy Selberg
Age 91
Rogers, AR

Dear Sayre:

So you want to know how I lived to be so old and still have my zip? *Enthusiastic positive thinking*.

Enthusiasm is catching. Think positive and good things happen. My gift shop on Cape Cod once attracted customers such as Jackie Kennedy. Today I drive a little white sports car and I'm still in business.

My wheeling and dealing continues in Arkansas as an antique and auction expert. A newspaper article about my positive thinking attitude decorates the lobby of the flea market where I have a booth. People come from all over to browse "Trudy's Treasures."

When I met the president of a large food company, I enthusiastically told him he needed me to help sell his products. Result: I'm the "granny" who removes his pies from the oven on television commercials.

Notice my letterhead. Fido was my theme at my 90th birthday. He'll oversee my "surprise" party when I'm 100. Who says an old dog can't look forward and plan ahead?

Enthusiastic positive thinking. Want to know what I'm wearing to the Healthy Aging awards ceremony at the Smithsonian in May? Guess.

Love,
Auntie Trudy

CALIFORNIA

Helen Quackenbush
Age 100
North Hollywood, CA

I am 100 years old and still going strong! I live in my own home and still exercise daily by walking three times around my badminton court, three times a day. I still drink a martini when out for dinner, and no one can tell me I won't live longer for not eating my vegetables . . . I never did like them. Young people today need to take time for themselves. If you are not happy with yourself, you can't be as healthy as possible. I've lived with love, family, God, and my country. I've lived and grown with my children and grandchildren, been there for them when they needed me, and waited on the sidelines while they learned from their own mistakes. I know I grew stronger from each experience, and I believe they did too. Through all these years, happiness seemed to help bring me good health. My belief is being happy is healthy and with good health you have a solid rock for your life's foundation.

COLORADO

Jessie Wakefield
Age 91+
Denver, CO

To Whom it May Concern:

Now that I have reached the age of 91+, I have determined that if a person wants to accomplish Healthy Aging one should:

Physically: Never smoke or drink; use plenty of apple cider vinegar, honey, and garlic; and take a nap whenever possible.

Socially: Love many and trust few.

Mentally: Think pleasant thoughts and never say anything bad about your fellow man.

Financially: Never carry a credit card or borrow money.

CONNECTICUT

Ann Capriola
Age 98
Norwalk, CT

My name is Ann Capriola and I am 98 years old. I owe my good health and long living to the fact that I started taking walks at a very young age and never stopped walking until recently. Dad and I would have our daily walk after dinner every day. When I married and the children came I would walk to school with one in a baby carriage and the others walking themselves. I would walk over two miles a day to go shopping and another two miles to get back home.

I have always liked to cook and bake, and I did a lot of it. Once I made 27 pies in one day! I still bake occasionally. For my birthday this year I am going to make a large Italian sponge cake topped with whipped cream, cherries, and walnuts.

I still have a very good memory. I have always liked to read history and trivia, and still do. Later, I memorize the facts and practice them which keeps my memory functioning. Besides reading, I write to family and friends.

FLORIDA

Kathryn Zane
Age 100
Anthony, FL

Age is nothing but numbers; and how you think will determine how you feel.

Take it from me, the youngest of nine children who rode a horse back and forth to be educated in a one-room school, and who spans time travel from the horse and buggy to computerized autos and jet airliners—you must believe all things are possible and work together for good!

Preserve your healthy balance of normal function by eating regular meals including plenty of fruits and vegetables. Follow a discipline of walking—not riding—use the stairs—not the elevator—and use your brain, not a calculator.

Never hold a grudge and stay away from medicines!

GEORGIA

Jane J. Allen
Age 91+
Atlanta, GA

Listening to a Sunday morning sermon by Dr. W. Frank Harrington, minister of the Peachtree Presbyterian Church of Atlanta, Georgia, I heard the word that would express my thoughts on Healthy Aging. It was taken from the Scripture verse in Philippians 4-10-18: "... for I have learned how to get along, happily, whether I have much or little ... I have learned the secret of *contentment* in every situation ..." I have found that this and an optimistic attitude can contribute to good health and a long life—91-plus years.

Experiencing the Great Depression taught us many things. Our values changed. Not only did we lose our jobs, and possessions, but we, personally, lost our two-year-old daughter. That is when we realized the importance of loved ones, friends, and the church.

Healthwise, there was no overindulgence in food, drink, or activities to injure our health.

I ended my active life as secretary to a vice president of a well known company. Now, I am living independently in a HUD subsidized senior citizen apartment complex, happy to be alive with my adoring family of a son, a daughter, five grandchildren and four great grandchildren. What more do I need for a healthy, happy, contented long life?

ILLINOIS

Ann L. Mendelsohn
Age 90+
Chicago, IL

I am 90+ (4-01-03) facing life changes so that it is not a struggle. I try to work at living each day in a state of "spark." Having had triple bypass surgery in 1992, exercising became a must. I exercise daily, at the same time and the same place. Later in the day I walk tall (or not at all!). I have an occasional body massage and visit doctors when required.

My memory is slipping in remembering—"What's his name . . . I know him," "Where did I put it?" etc. I am now writing things down. When eating in restaurants, for weight control I request half orders and go easy on the fats and sugar. I enjoy reading, theater, movies, lectures, and being with younger folks.

I was a guest at the Chicago Senior Olympics recently and I am looking forward to 1997 to qualify for the 12K walk. Daily I relax and repeat the following meditation, "I am an open channel through which the healing currents of God are now flowing. Spirit is my life, my health, my supply, and my prosperity."

Now I am looking forward to at least an additional seven years of living with new interests. I have much love to give and to receive.

INDIANA

Mazo Modesitt
Age 91
Brazil, IN

Reaching the golden years is a challenge, a blessing, an opportunity, and a gift from God. It behooves each of us to live with a desire to make each day a happier and more wholesome environment for everyone, from the babe in the cradle to the little lady in her wheelchair.

Look around friend—get rid of your negative attitude. Lend a helping hand to someone less fortunate, a word of encouragement to someone depressed. Forget self and look beyond your limitations by helping someone enjoy a brighter tomorrow, and thus bringing a glow to your life.

Sure we have our moments when we ask ourselves, "What am I doing here?" It's up to us to find the answer. You may throw up your hands in despair or gird yourself with determination to make the most of your golden years.

Think of the little neglected child whom others shun because of physical defects. Give him a cookie, read him a story. You may help change his entire life. So many opportunities to use our talents. What are we waiting for? Let's get busy today.

IOWA

Florence Collins
Age 98
Mt. Pleasant, IA

Dear Future Generations of America:

I was born on a Henry County, Iowa farm, December 28, 1897, where I enjoyed good food, water, clean fresh air, and plenty of exercise.

After attending Howe's Academy, I obtained my first teacher's certificate. I continued teaching and attending Iowa Wesleyan College until graduating Magna Cum Laude in 1929. I retired after 30 years of teaching.

My father, his mother, and several siblings lived past 80. One sister reached 90; another sister and a brother nearly 100. My living sister is nearly 95.

I was 87-plus when a malignant kidney was removed. As I went into surgery the scripture, "I will trust and not be afraid," sustained me. At 97, failing eyesight caused me to give up driving.

I believe the reason I am having a long life is because God has willed it to be so, and is taking care of me.

Perhaps you didn't have a good start. Any hope for you? Yes, turn your life over to God who can yet make something beautiful of it. Then whether your life be long or short, all will be well. It is eternity that counts!

KANSAS

Frank Brady
Age 93
Frankfort, KS

Letter to Future Generations:

I am 93 years young so I feel qualified to give you some advice on Healthy Aging. I was born in 1903 and attended the St. Louis World's Fair in 1904. Because I am in excellent health, I will comment on what has worked for me, both with regard to my physical health and my financial health.

I have been a farmer all my life and firmly believe "hard work," specifically physical labor, is the key to good physical health. Besides engaging in vigorous exercise every day, another thing I have done *every* day of my life is eat a "good" breakfast. A good breakfast is essential for a good day's work! Another thing I strive for each day is a nap. Even if it's only a 20- or 30-minute nap, I awaken feeling totally energized.

I believe in a strong work ethic. I always gave an honest day's work for an honest day's pay. My philosophy is "it's not how much you make but how you *manage* what you make." This belief has enabled me to be financially healthy.

P.S. If it wasn't time for breakfast now, I'd give you more advice!

LOUISIANA

Gibbs D. Miller, Sr.
Age 93
Vinton, LA

My name is Gibbs D. Miller. I am 93 years old. I was born in 1903 and have been married for 68 years. I've lived through two world wars, the Depression, and have seen the Berlin Wall go up and come down. I guess if I have any age old wisdom to share it would be about staying mentally fit. At my age your mental health is most important. Keeping my mind sharp keeps me young. I feel that if I don't do things that stimulate me or challenge me mentally, I would probably go down quickly. I feel this is vitally important for my age group and have observed this to be true with my friends and loved ones. This is easily achieved. Besides reading the paper and newsletters, one of the things I do to stay mentally fit is that I play the card game solitaire every night. I feel it keeps me going and presents a mental challenge for me too. Equally important, I walk and also eat a hearty breakfast of bacon, eggs, toast, milk, juice, and coffee *every* morning. I have never missed my breakfast in 93 years.

MARYLAND

Sirarpi Khoyan
Age 92
Chevy Chase, MD

I hope my life will be an inspiration to the new generation—systematic 15-minute calisthenics and three-mile walks every day, rain or shine.

After college and two years of medical school, I continued my education by reading books, newspapers, and keeping an interest in current events. Instead of stagnating with people my own age, I enjoyed younger people. I kept myself mentally young by helping and getting involved with their lives. After raising three children, I started working at age 54. I looked 20 years younger because I never smoked or indulged in alcoholic beverages. I took pride in my appearance. At 85, I retired.

Seven years ago, my husband passed away. I was totally lost. I felt sick and despondent and wanted to die. I had headaches and could not sleep. My granddaughter encouraged me to write my life history. I wrote 500 pages and gave copies to my children and grandchildren.

Today, I am 92 years old. I exercise. I still walk three miles a day. I have joined church groups. I read and lecture. I take pleasure in group vacations and instead of wanting to die, I have learned to give thanks to my God.

MASSACHUSETTS

Charles W. Farrington
Age 93
Bedford, MA

To a Young American:

Although you enjoy youth while I am nearly 94, we both possess a mystical inner power. It is always there for consultation and guidance. May it guide you through a long and happy life. You are an American, where the only dictator is your own conscience. You own a working share in its future. Encouragement comes from Shakespeare's *Hamlet*; "To thine own self be true . . ." and Ralph Waldo Emerson's "Trust thyself, every heart vibrates to that iron string."

You enter a world made closer by fast air travel, orbiting surveillance, and instantaneous worldwide communication. Also a world adjusting to a building human population. As you also adjust to the rapid rate of change, find the rewards of moderation in everything you do. Make music part of your life. Songs you hear during romantic years linger long, mingling with fond memories. Discover the lasting melodies of Beethoven's Pastoral ride into the country in spring. Enjoy happy "Pops" music, Ragtime, lively Sousa marches. Thrill to a muleback ride down the sheer wall of the Grand Canyon. I wish you a long and happy life!

MICHIGAN

Frank Jacobson
Age 90
Dearborn Heights, MI

Dear Martin:

Thank you for the great card you sent me for my 90th birthday a couple of weeks ago. Just think, I'm *ten times* as old as you! At your age you can never believe you will be 90 years old, but if you watch your health, you might make it. My advice is, get a lot of exercise. When I was a boy there were few cars, my folks were too poor to keep a horse or to buy me a bike, so I did a lot of walking. When the Higgens Lake froze over in winter my brother and I skated across to school, otherwise we skied or walked around.

The school was just one room, one teacher, and children in all eight grades. I was in fourth grade, and had to take my turn fetching in wood for the big pot belly stove. It is a long way from that school to computers. At home we had to carry in wood and haul out the ashes. There was no TV or even radio. I owe my long years to getting plenty of exercise, so keep active, Martin, and God bless you.

Love,
Grandpa Frank

MINNESOTA

Gunnel Johnson
Age 96$\frac{1}{2}$
Minneapolis, MN

I am now 96$\frac{1}{2}$ years old—though I do not feel that old. I am now walking to the bus, going downtown to do my errands. I gave up my car at age 92. I still live in the house my husband bought in 1927 in the beautiful city of Minneapolis, Minnesota, with beautiful lakes and parks. My husband, who died 22 years ago, and I were always traveling to foreign countries and all over the U.S.A.

I believe that my enthusiasm, stamina and love of life has kept me independent to continue to live in my own home and travel to visit my large family, settled in the country. I love to read, watch, and keep up with the news and write letters. Do not give up what you can still do by yourself, but accept favors and help from friends and family gratefully.

MISSISSIPPI

Luna W. Clay
Age 92
Waynesboro, MS

My advice to the future generations on how to live a long, healthy, happy, and useful life is you should be very aware of the importance of maintaining a healthy body and a happy mental attitude.

I would advise you to eat nutritious food and take plenty of physical exercise into the 90s.

Keep a happy mental attitude by seeking new knowledge through reading and associating with interesting people for new ideas. This will enhance the quality of living. Continue to appreciate and enjoy the gifts of life, such as family, friends, and the privilege of spiritual communication.

Guard your thoughts and keep them in the right channels. Remember the quotation: "As a man thinketh, so is he."

MISSOURI

Constance Vulliamy
Age 90
Parkville, MO

The process of aging begins when we are born and continues throughout life! In addition to the basic things like not smoking or taking drugs, there are some things I have found very worthwhile—moderation in eating for instance, and a reasonable amount of exercise and sleep.

I have enjoyed reading, rather than too much TV. Also mobility, including driving even if limited, and a reasonably good education, also whatever travel can be managed. They both help extend one's interests in what is going on in the world, and add to enjoyment of different people, places, and things.

Basic to everything is good health, including eyesight.

An optimistic outlook on life not only makes living more satisfying, but also affects one's health, I think.

There are, however, some things over which one has no control, and which are in fact just pure luck! It is, for instance, good to have healthy parents, physically, mentally, and spiritually. These I had, which made for a happy childhood, despite lack of money.

I also feel that work is a real blessing, including volunteer work after retirement. Finally, when feeling lonely, it helps to make the effort to help someone else.

MONTANA

William D. Cane
Age 90
Great Falls, MT

I am an extremely active 90, still passionate and alert, caring for all personal needs, living alone in a thirty by sixty foot house, driving my car, and caring for my financial affairs, which require close attention to detail. For years, I have prepared breakfast, consisting of dry whole grain cereals with milk, (no sugar) juice, fruit, whole wheat toast (no coffee). I do drink two or three cups throughout the day. Other meals, I eat out. I have always eaten at regular intervals, morning, noon, and early evening. I hardly ever snacked. I still have my own teeth. My life work has been principally a musician; performing, teaching, and composing. I have also been a radio announcer, salesman, and landlord. But music has always been there in one form or another. I still perform occasionally, still compose, and vocalize—especially teach saxophone, clarinet, flute, guitar, and banjo.

I dance (and very energetically) two or three times a week, totaling about 12 hours of exercise.

I am not sure why I have retained so much energy and ability at my age, but I believe it is mostly due to loving my work and continuing to do it.

NEVADA

Ruth DeHan
Age 91
Las Vegas, NV

Dear Contest Judges:

I am 91 years of age and for the past fifteen years have been a volunteer with the Retired Senior Volunteer Program in various programs, seven of which I was the volunteer coordinator.

I have discovered that volunteering is a great healer. I moved to Las Vegas the latter part of 1981, after the death of my husband; our happy marriage lasted 48 years. At that time, my oldest daughter joined me in Las Vegas (I have since lost her to leukemia). I needed some way to recover somewhat from my losses. Frankly, as a volunteer, I was able to "do some good," as evidenced by the many awards that I've received over the years—but in all honesty, volunteering has given me a great deal more than I have given.

I still do volunteer work for the Retired Senior Volunteer Program and have just undertaken a volunteer clerical assignment with the Respite Care Referral Service program. I still need that "lifeline" of volunteering.

NEW HAMPSHIRE

Edith B. Cheever
Age 91
Nashua, NH

Dear Adult 50-plus:

As part of the National Healthy Aging Campaign, I am writing this letter to you to encourage you to develop a positive attitude for growing older.

I am now a widow in my 90s-plus. I am in good health and enjoy each day. Maybe you can benefit by knowing how I am living these later years in a retired community. I had many interests which I could not follow earlier because I was busy caring for my family. Now I lead a group of 30 ladies in knitting for needy children. This has opened my world to many interesting people and for which I have received surprising rewards.

On my 90th birthday I presented each of my three adult children with a book of memoirs in which I had written some stories of my youth for them. What a treasure!

I did not drink or smoke, ate a well-balanced diet, and always have had plenty of exercise and rest. I have periodic checks with my doctor, but avoid medication when possible.

I hope you will find my way of life helpful in your living long and happily.

Your 90-plus friend.

NEW JERSEY

Lillian Grunt
Age 91
South Orange, NJ

How to grow old gracefully.

Since I have reached the age of 91, I ponder on what wisdom I have gathered to sustain me. I find that life is a learning process, and I have grown spiritually and naturally. While overcoming many obstacles, I found it brought me to an understanding of what problems growth can give me. While I live alone, I am not lonely, since my spiritual growth has enhanced my knowledge. I have a scrapbook of things and ideas that I collected, some I wrote, and also in my reading on the great mystic and great philosophies. I read them when companionship is not available, since most of my friends and family are gone. It is something I cherish. I take courses at universities and read good literature. Having a positive attitude helps. Every day I try to help someone in need and indirectly this does much for me. I thank God for the blessings.

P.S. I still drive and go to the pool three times a week. I exercise and walk.

NEW YORK

Constance (Connie) Falconer
Age 92
Burnt Hills, NY

Hi!

The single most important thing I have learned about Healthy Aging is twofold:

1. Keep moving and
2. Eat plenty of fruit, particularly apples.

My husband, a civil engineer building roads and bridges, bought land and planted an apple orchard as a side line. I toted boxes and bags of apples for 30 years. Hence, I ate many apples, and still do, core and all!

Now I run a B & B business—my laundry is 11 steps down. My second floor, on which I house my Bed and Breakfast guests, is 15 steps up, 26 steps in all, which I traverse many times a day. (I do all the laundry. My household helper comes three hours one day every two weeks.) Keeping moving has kept my weight down, my knees limber, and my back straight.

At 92 I can still kneel in church, weed my garden on all fours, play bridge every Wednesday night, and drive my car during the daylight hours.

I think this is under 200 words and I have certainly said enough.

NORTH CAROLINA

Louise Randel
Age 100
Hendersonville, NC

I was 100 on March 29, 1996. I never thought about it, but I was amazed how much 100 meant to others. The parties, gifts, and cards overwhelmed me and I personally wrote to those who so kindly remembered me—two hundred individuals and four organizations to which I belong.

I have enjoyed good health and I have not abused my body in any way. I have always kept active. That is most essential, especially after retirement. There is much to be done in all fields of endeavor and volunteers are needed. I have followed my advice and am still helping children in school who have difficulty in reading. I also teach folks from Japan to speak English. It is a gratifying experience.

NORTH DAKOTA

Ben Walsh
Age 97
Fargo, ND

In order to conduct a contest such as you are doing, it is understandable that you know a person's age, physical, and mental condition. Well, here is mine in a brief, but easily understood form:

I am 97 years of age, having been born in a homestead shack in the heart of a Dakota winter. Physically I am very well indeed, considering my age. I walk two miles each day, rain or shine, outside when the weather is fit, and inside when it is not. I have a hearty appetite. I eat three square meals each day. My mind is as sharp as it has always been.

I attribute my good health (both physical and mental) to the fact that I have always led a clean and healthy life. I have never abused my good health by pouring liquor into it. I have always lived a sober, sensible life, and I feel that now I am being repaid for the clean life that I have led. My example should be a good example for the youth of today.

OHIO

Lonnie Stewart
Age 105
Cincinnati, OH

Dear Future Generations:

I am 105 years old. I have lived to get old, but it is only through the grace of God. If you want to live a long time, you've got to put your faith in God. You've got to treat everybody right. I grew up on a farm. I was a sharecropper. I had a wife and eight children. Six children are still living. My wife lived to be 84. I live with my daughter now.

I always read my Bible and pray every day. My eyes are not as good as they used to be, but I still go to church. I still like to discuss the Bible.

You have to be honest. You have to treat everyone exactly the same way you want to be treated.

Pray every day and take care of yourself. Stay busy, it will help your mind. Don't ever forget about God.

OKLAHOMA

Lois S. Millerborg
Age 92
Oklahoma City, OK

I was born into a large family. A great training preparation for life.

At six I was playing outside. Annie worked for us. She saw me fall and could see I was not hurt. She called to me, "Lois come here and I'll pick you up." She loved me, sent me back to my play. When I got to the corner of the house, I looked back and said, "Annie didn't pick me up, I picked myself up." That lesson taught me a lot.

Started a nursing career at 55. Served on the first open-heart team here.

At 65, successfully operated a resale shop for 13 years.

Teach your children to work. They will hate you if you don't. We taught ours and loved them. Married 58 challenging years.

Don't allow people to over lean on you. This breeds weaklings.

Always be good to yourself. Eat wholesome food. Keep well, exercise, and rest.

Stay out of debt or you will be a slave to your debtor.

Enjoy fellowship with your fellow man. Listen part of the time.

Be honest, you will sleep better.

Glorify God, you will be blessed.

OREGON

Elsie Davidson Carr
Age 90
Corvallis, OR

My Dear Great-grandchildren:

If there is any legacy I could leave to you it would be this: Have faith in God and be thankful! You helped me celebrate my wonderful ninetieth birthday. You know how much I enjoy life and appreciate the love of my family and many friends.

When I was small I was taught the "Golden Rule" so I believe in the Law of Reciprocity. If I give a smile, I get one back. If I do a kind deed, it returns two-fold or more. I treat my body well by giving it pleasant exercise, good nutritious food, and peaceful rest. I don't mistreat it with tobacco, drugs, or alcohol. It repays me with good health. When my soul and spirit are happy—my body is happy! "He who lives well lives long."

And I am so grateful for everything I have! I don't forget to say "thank you" over and over. You know I have lived on three continents but I am proudly thankful to live in America. I've learned that trusting God and having an *attitude of gratitude* pays off in gracious living and healthy longevity.

With my love and prayers,
Your Great-grandma

PENNSYLVANIA

Marjorie G. Ruch
Age 91
Lancaster, PA

Dear Youthful Friends:

The single most important thing that helped me reach healthful aging was the ability with a little luck to make the best choices. This was aided by education, helpful friends, and deliberation.

My parents were healthy people and luckily gave me some health-promoting genes. Now I had to maintain a healthy body and soul.

For body help, I chose to eat nourishing food and to exercise. I started exercising early in life, before I started to fall apart. I chose individual sports, such as golf, tennis, and swimming—which I could enjoy, and joined exercise classes.

Wise choices for the soul can be helped by choosing a good faith, which teaches love through consideration and helpfulness for others. Don't forget to pray—anytime, anyplace.

I believe the two biggest choices in life are choosing a vocation — what should I do with my life and choosing a mate, if that is your desire. Both choices require a great deal of thoughtful decision. Do all you can to get the knowledge, advice, and background to help you make the right choices.

I enclose my best wishes to you for making these choices.

TENNESSEE

Chris P. Keim
Age 90½
Oak Ridge, TN

As I looked ahead to retirement 25 years ago, my principal interrelated personal concerns were health, finances, activities, and attitudes.

Among those, good health has been most important because it has allowed me to stay active.

At retirement the best choice I made was to reaffirm my commitment to regular exercise. I walk, row, lift weights, and use nautilus machines.

I am also concerned with what I eat, drink, and breathe.

My good health has enabled me to participate in interesting activities. I have worked with small colleges and in the space program. I acquired my private pilot certificate. I have been active in community organizations.

One of my exercise and recreation pastimes has been rowing. I became a certified judge-referee for regattas. I developed rowing programs for the physically disabled and the mentally retarded.

Good health has aided my wife and me with our other concerns. Our finances are under control. Our expenditures are less than our income. We have sufficient insurance. We have a reserve for emergencies. We have no indebtedness.

Positive attitudes and a strong faith are vital. We are fortunate in retirement. The choices we made early in our retirement have played a large part.

TEXAS

Gladys Casimir
Age 95
Calvert, TX

Dear Future Youth of America:

I would like to challenge you to prepare yourselves for the coming century. With 95 years of living experience, I want to share with you my secret for healthy aging.

Have you ever heard the saying, "My mind to me a kingdom is?" I have found my own mind to be a kingdom, and I have sought constantly to keep it agile, flexible, and creative. My "mind kingdom" has empowered me to make good choices, enjoy an independent and productive life, and to follow a daily routine that pleases and sustains me.

Today I am able to maintain my own home, teach my women's weekly Sunday School class, and worship in my church on Sundays and Wednesdays. I enjoy reading the Bible, books about Texas history, and other subjects. I recently proofread chapters of a manuscript, presented a Royal Service program, and conducted a book review. I also walk two miles a day when weather permits.

I encourage you to choose to discover your own "mind kingdom" and to begin developing the mental skills that will empower you to realize your dreams. May God bless each of you with a long and productive life in the 21st century.

UTAH

W. Le Grande Law
Age 98 + 10$\frac{1}{2}$ months
Delta, UT

Dear Future Generations of Americans:

Being a Veteran of World War I, I say to you: Love and protect our beautiful United States of America, and please remember that on November 11, 1918 at the 11th hour of the 11th day of the 11th month the Armistice was signed, ending World War I. It was to be the Great War to end all wars. Sadly, it wasn't.

I will be 99 on December 16, and I have some suggestions. Be the best person you can be. Have faith in God and in yourself. Give thanks for each day, and take care of yourselves—you just may live to be 100!

Eat good food. Find happiness in simple things like gardening and sharing your harvest with others. Learn the value of honest labor; make your word your bond. Be thrifty. Keep mentally and physically active with keen sense for learning.

Develop God-given talents—especially good music, the universal language that can bring inspiration and joy to the world. Don't use drugs or alcohol.

And most important: Pray for wisdom to make right choices and engender love and support in your families.

God bless you all.

VERMONT

Mildred Douglas Gibson
Age 93
Island Pond, VT

I'm enjoying being an active part of senior activities.

I do not act and feel old. Why should I?

I've led an active and happy life.

My whole life has included work activities.

During the eighth grade I was school janitor in a rural school district. I also trapped muskrats to earn money.

I worked for my board during high school and normal school. I taught school 34 years plus substituting and later teaching remedial reading.

My husband and I raised a son who is a commercial artist.

I won prizes in original cooking contests.

I'm past president of a Relief Corps, Woman's Club, and Retired Teachers Association. I was the Grange's musician.

I have been a church clerk and Sunday school teacher.

Now-a-days I live alone, write poetry, and am active in community life.

I'm healthy, active, and happy.

WASHINGTON

Miriam Snow Mathes
Age 91
Lacey, WA

How to live 91 years? Have an absorbing interest, preferably creative, challenging, inexpensive and unrelated to daily work. Mine has been writing—but not the great American novel!

Even before high school and college it was a page-a-day diary-keeping. Scribbling my discoveries in New York City kept homesickness at bay in my first position. Voluntary book reviewing and lighthearted professional articles followed. When traveling, nightly I recorded impressions, not information. Custom-made for the individual were Christmas letters, those of congratulations, sympathy, and just keeping in touch. Reward came 40 years ago on learning a young grandson slept with my latest under his pillow.

Now, while memories are still vivid, I reminisce: *Life on the Home Front During the 20th Century Wars*, 90 years of living, *Global Retirement* (vignettes of travel in the 1970s as *The Iron Curtain Rising*. Since my 90th birthday, 20 have been finished with titles for several more selected).

No readers? You might be surprised. I was. But the real satisfaction is the feeling of accomplishment. Incidentally, with practice, writing becomes easier, observation keener, recollection better. Written communication gives lasting pleasure and is tangible proof an oldster is still alert.

WEST VIRGINIA

Lucille B. Meredith
Age 92
Fairmont, WV

Focus on the positive! Do not dwell on the negative. Have a set of values which will serve as a compass when things are confusing.

Don't be afraid to take a calculated risk. Think twice, speak once.

Share your feelings with someone else—a friend or counselor.

The brain has some similarities to ordinary muscles and it must be exercised and used regularly to be able to perform at its best.

Use your mind. Challenge it and expose it to new ideas.

Read the kinds of things you haven't read before.

Write, for writing requires ordered thinking.

Volunteer or teach, when you teach you learn.

Play games that require thought like chess or bridge. Try to work a crossword puzzle a day.

Watch TV shows that challenge the intellect.

Remember to walk. It's good for the brain and the body.

Be an optimist. Don't tell your troubles. Eighty percent couldn't care less and 20% are glad to find someone more miserable than they are!

A smile is more important than your lipstick or your shaving lotion.

Live life every day as if it's your very last.

WISCONSIN

Vanita Volkert
Age 94
Madison, WI

My Dear Descendants:

What a privilege it is to write about Healthy Aging! It is a joy to recall the many good things (and sometimes less pleasing incidents) that befall one during a lifetime.

This time of the year, autumn, is the most colorful time of all seasons. The trees are donning their most gorgeous colors—yellow, orange, red, and brown. Petunias, marigolds, and chrysanthemums are vying with each other, in grandeur, before the first frost nips their beauty.

Life's autumn, the declining years, is similar to nature's pattern. The seeds of life's autumn are sown in the carefree days of childhood, in the fleeting years of youth, and through the busy years of adulthood. Seeds of love and understanding, seeds of honor, hope and perseverance, seeds of faith and integrity. We shall pass through life victoriously knowing we have left footprints worthy of our posterity to follow.

Experience has taught us that if we desire to reap the harvest of a full, meaningful life we must conform to healthy living habits. It is our duty to choose health-giving foods; to practice proper living habits; and to "take time to smell the roses."

WYOMING

Dolores Brady
Age 90
Gillette, WY

I would like to see the young people of today live by the saving method instead of buying on credit.

If they would save a small amount of their paychecks each month, over a lifetime it will double and triple many times. At retirement their nest egg would be large, also still making money.

Invest your money in different things such as real estate, bonds, mutual funds, etc.

Learning to manage when young is so important, that pattern stays with you through the years. You lose temptation to spend and enjoy seeing your money grow.

If a person buys on credit you pay the purchase price plus interest on the credit, which amounts to paying twice. Only buy what you need. Think before you buy; do I really need this many things? You do not! Let's eliminate the worry and stress of debt.

Money is funny, it grows without sunshine, air, water, or soil. Just keep it invested.

As we turn the pages of time we find more wisdom comes with each day. Use it managing your money as you travel through life.

More Gems of Wisdom

Thousands of letters were written by Americans. Although it was difficult to choose five winners from each state and Washington, DC, we also felt there were so many other wonderful letters to share. Following are quotes and excerpts from some of our favorite non-winning leters, offering each writer's secrets for Healthy Aging...

As for mental health, when I'm depressed I put on some *loud* Rock & Roll, Good Blues and dance alone. It's good for your heart rate.
— *Jean Barchanowicz, age 54, Pine Level, AL*

Eating prunes for both young and old is part of the learning of regularity.
— *Frank Thomas, age 72, Birmingham, AL*

Just recently, a four-year-old said to my wife, "You have an old neck." Out of the mouths of babes... but it is a funny fact of life...Make memories for tomorrow and thank God for your old neck.
— *Hank Nelson, 63, Craig, AK*

This much I know, every time I smile and throw my shoulders back, I feel better about myself and the world around me. And who knows how many visits to the doctor I have saved by smiling and standing tall. Try it when you feel low.
— *Gary Bousman, 85, Phoenix, AZ*

Age is simply a number. Numbers have the meaning that we assign to them. If age were the determinant of health, all people of the same age would be exactly alike by all health standards. But we know that is not true.
— *Norma Richardson, 72, Tucson, AZ*

Dream! If your life has been stale and dull, change it...Respect yourself. Unless it happens to be truly rewarding to live to serve others, be selfish enough to do things that have meaning for you. Learn to recognize things that make you feel sorry for yourself and avoid them.
— *Ann Wynngate, 77, Fayetteville, AR*

Let me share with you a wonderful habit I have acquired over the years. Just before going to sleep at night, think of the best thing that happened to you that particular day. You'll be guaranteed a restful night's sleep if you practice this "happy thought of the day" trick.
— *Joan Wimberly, 62, Fayetteville, AR*

Blindness while trying to excel in varied fields of endeavors may seem to be an antithesis to visualization. But nothing could be further from the truth. I made the best weight throws while being blind. Why? Because I could not see the end result, but concentrated on what it took to do my best. Don't quit whatever is good in life.
— *Bill Bangert, 72, Anaheim, CA*

While my suggestions for Healthy Aging may not be profound or difficult to follow, I hope some readers might live by a motto I try to be mindful of each morning: "Today is a gift—that is why it is called the present."
— *Blanche E. Wilson, 89, Claremont, CA*

Here are the guide-posts of my life: 1. Learn to accept what cannot be changed. 2. See beauty in each person, each day. 3. Laugh—see humor in unusual circumstances. 4. Express love and accept in return. 5. Exercise your mind and body daily. 6. Develop a lively imagination. 7. Volunteer expecting no repayment.
— *Nora G. Hecker, 87, Sherman Oaks, CA*

Count your blessings. My daughter's friend has cerebral palsy. Her walk is awkward, her speech slurred. But she just completed college and is optimistically looking for a job. She recently told me, "I'm luckier than lots of people. I could be paralyzed." When change happens, consider and be grateful for what you have.
— *Barbara L. Arn, 71, Arcadia, CA*

Stay relaxed and serene. Avoid loud, vulgar, selfish, humorless, insensitive people. Allow others to be who they have to be. Try not to fear for them or take on their pain. Appreciate the beauty in everyone. Enjoy what you have. Give no thought to "what could have been."
— *Val Croll, 69, Steamboat Springs, CO*

When people volunteer loving attention to young people, the rewards to each are very uplifting and promote a high level of social health. A youthful spirit it something that can endure until death. What a gain!
— *Sharon Thorvaldson, 52, Longmont, CO*

I commented to the doctor that he must be doing very well for himself based on the number of folks sitting there waiting to see him. He told me only half of the people sitting there were waiting to see him. The rest were friends. The key, he told me, to living long and well was to have a friend. This could be a spouse, a buddy, heck it could be a dog or cat. The important thing was to have someone or something to care about, who cared about you, and then you have the key to successful aging.
— *Thomas McMullen, 54, Newington, CT*

There is an old axiom "It takes more muscles to frown than to smile." So, future generations, remember the smile, the busy-bee attitude (never give up), and keep the faith that makes it all worthwhile.
— *Doris Perdue, 72, Lewes, DE*

Letter writing is the salvation of we older folks. As we age and go far beyond retirement there is nothing more depressing than an empty mailbox. So to you young folks growing up and older I say cultivate communicating by letter. It will pay great dividends in your later years.
— *Ted Ressler, 70, Camden, DE*

Some secrets of old age: Do not argue with yourself everyday. . .Your stomach is not a garbage can.
— *Max Fleisher, 93 1/2, N. Miami Beach, FL*

I ride my exercycle every morning and swim every afternoon.
— *Rhoda Kuster, 92, Winter Haven, FL*

If you can't do physical exercise, exercise your brain!
— *Anne D. Soule, 90, Miami, FL*

My advice—love God and people, owe no man, eat well, sleep well, and keep a Yorkie puppy by your side.
— *Elizabeth S. Anderson, 84, Milton, FL*

There's a train called Life passing by and we can get on for the ride or we can miss it... Talk with a cow, rub a dog's ears, listen to a child, and lie in the grass and consider the stars. . .And, it's only just begun, for there's a train a'comin'!
— *Ted Brooke, 53, Cumming, GA*

Any worries you may have—save them all and plan a "worry day." Pick a time when you will attend to them all at once. Any that are left over after half a day—tie them in for the next "worry day."
— *Carolyn L. Falk, 76, Eastanolle, GA*

Never stop growing and learning. Always do your very best and look forward to the next challenge; good *intentions* aren't good enough. Rarely quit. Maintain a great sense of humor. Appreciate love and beauty in all their forms.
— *E. Milton Wilson, 68, Honolulu, HI*

Live below your finances so that you can save or invest at least 10% of your income. Have a nest egg of at least three months of living expenses before you begin investing.
— *Michael F. Henely, 73, Honolulu, HI*

Above all I learned that life is not perfect, but it does have its rewards if you listen and learn before it is too late.
— *Edward Greenberg, 81, Chelsea, MA*

A healthy retirement (package) does you no good if you are not alive—wealth without health is of very little value.
— *Marilyn Watts, 65, Idaho Falls, ID*

As a physician, my impression is that those who look young have something they look forward to doing each day. It may be golf or grandchildren, swimming or shuffleboard, cruises or crocheting, but it occupies their minds and often their bodies as well.
— *L. D. Gilley, M.D., 58, Newburgh, IN*

Keep learning. . . wear bright colors. . . Smile!
— *Mary E. Risch, 80, Connersville, IN*

If I have learned anything, it is that we are the drum major in our parade of life.
— *Marion S. Clark, 72, Cedar Falls, IA*

Healthy Aging isn't a gift you receive along with a gold watch and your walking papers. It is acquired through a lifetime of caring about and for yourself.
— *Ramona Morse, 71, Osage, IA*

My philosophy for my aging years is "I may be getting old, but I refuse to grow up." If I can maintain my childhood love, trust, and wonder I'll be young forever, even though I am almost 85 years old.
— *Elaine Hayden, 84 + 10 mo., Edgerton, KS*

I love to write letters, send cards, remember birthdays, and I send 200 Christmas cards. Telephones are great, but seeing things is much better. I'm often kidded about my letter writing, but I just consider the source and laugh.
— *Julia Rowand, 77, Danville, KY*

But one must strive, in life's decline
To wear one's age like vintage wine.
— *Beverly L. Tagge, 70, Baton Rouge, LA*

Exercise at least every other day by brisk walking for a mile or two; compete in organized sports like Senior Olympics. Do this and you will feel better physically, mentally, and younger in spirit.
— *Frank E. Herrelko, Sr., 83, Bowie, MD*

There is no replay in life. . .This is it.
— *Dorothea Frysingera, 80, Boothbay, ME*

Fear not the changes. You have a jump start over your forbearers: you are taller, stronger, faster than they; your access to the world's increasing knowledge is instantaneous and sophisticated; you will, I feel sure, embrace the elimination of discrimination in all its forms; you recognize that money is but one of life's many satisfactions.
— *Alec Dyson Brown, 80, Fall River, MA*

Don't say, "In my day" as if the day is over. If you are still here to say it, then today is your day. You are part of these tumultuous, exciting, stimulating days. Grab them, cherish them, Don't say, "In my day." Instead say, "Here and now—these are my days, every single one of them."
— *Helen G. Purcell, 77, Wellfleet, MA*

Baby boomers, forget about your wrinkles and go out and cultivate a garden. To watch your garden grow and bloom will be an endless delight, and when your garden bears fruit, it will prove to be a most rewarding experience. After 40, every person paints his own portrait. Think happy thoughts and your portrait will be a pleasing and happy one.
— *Lillian Kline, 96, Worcester, MA*

Don't wait until retirement to acquire a variety of interests. Listening and participating in music is forever rewarding. Read the sports pages, follow a team. Politics can be interesting. Reading—especially biographies—is interesting.
— *Marguerite Smith, 91, Midland, MI*

I remain fit because I feel that the greatest gift I can give to my children is to be a *role model*, to continue my active prevention fitness routine that enables me to have the energy and good health to enjoy participating in their lives. . .Most important, *I do not want my family to be my caretaker.*
— *Catti Watson, 63, Chicago, IL*

In looking back on my life of 87 years, I can appreciate how many more educational opportunities are available today than when I was young. Look for diverse experiences, ask questions, listen to all people, young and old, develop a passion for reading, and always, always keep an open mind. I believe that education is knowledge and knowledge is power.
 — *Lillian La Rosa, 87, Wellesley, MA*

Trying something new is the single most important thing I have learned about Healthy Aging.
 — *Nadine Brockway, 53, Lake St. Louis, MO*

The secret to successful aging is...the need to belong, the need to be needed, and the need for security. That's why, at age 70, we're still making plans for the future.
 — *Bernelda V. Becker, 70, St. Louis Park, MN*

My husband is severely disabled, but we have traveled all over the world. Yes, it takes intense planning and determination, but it gives us something to look forward to, and where there's a will, there's a way. We have inspired other handicapped people to "go for it."
 — *Grace Hawkins, 69, Anoka, MN*

I discovered this gem from a Norwegian song that I would like to share with future generations: "La oss leve for hverandre og ta vare pa den tid vi har." Translated literally it means to live for each other and take care of the time we have.
 — *Clarice Anderson, 64, Minneapolis, MN*

For the first time in history we are a nation of people capable of building a free social order, seeking our own way toward happiness and mental well-being, forging some semblance of financial health, and lastly, making enlightened decisions about our lifestyles which will garner for us the full measure of years our Creator has allotted to us.
 — *Ronald L. Struwe, 70, Eden Prairie, MN*

Get out of bed each morning with the determination to be happy. The only force we can totally control is our attitude.
 — *Jocleta C. Cartledge, 58, Kitmichael, MS*

The "Clock of Life" is wound but once,
and no one has the power to tell
just when the hand will stop.
Now is the only time you own,
Live, Love, Toil with a will,
Place no faith in tomorrow,
The clock then may be still.
 — *Josephine G. Morrow, 80, Macon, MO*

Get outdoors! Ride a bicycle or walk on errands instead of driving a car. Feel the wind of the world on your face.
 — *Tom Eaton, 56, Kansas City, MO*

Relax!
> — *Dorothy Guice, 78, Jackson, MS*

Twenty-four years ago, soon after your father died, a wise friend gave me a sampler which she had beautifully embroidered and framed. It read, "The most wasted day of all is that on which you have not laughed."
> — *Mildred Miller, 76, Minneapolis, MN*

You wanted to know what we have learned in raising ten children and 46 grandchildren: pride, honesty, hospitality.
> — *Ruth Dahl, 68, Alden, MT*

The key to Healthy Aging is a sense of humor.
> — *Carla Kaufman, 58, Albion, NE*

Healthy Aging starts long before you reach "Senior Citizen" status. If you live your life in a positive way, achieving "Healthy Aging" will come as naturally as breathing.
> — *Helen Seymour, 66, Lincoln, NE*

To enjoy the embrace of your lover, to always kiss goodnight, to feel their admiring eyes on you as you meet in a restaurant, these things and more help keep one young.
> — *Joan S. Weinberger, 56, NV*

I never drank alcohol or smoked. And I cooked plain meals. I never went jogging for my exercise, I washed clothes with the washing board. There were no washers then.
> — *Carmela Di Cianno, 86, Ely, NV*

"Healthy" is measured not in blood pressure or heartbeats per minute but in love and wisdom, in caring about others, and taking care of yourself. It's in the way you look at life and the way you live your life, either straight on with a smile and a get-things-done spirit or with a sneer and an it's-good-enough approach. The choice is always yours.
> — *Mark Howat, 66, Surf City, NJ*

Give of your self, leave a legacy, a piece of work, a poem, a fishing trip, a memory, a "delight." My goal is to leave at least one each month. This is my gift to me, then returned to me no less than twelve encounters a year. And so I am building a tradition.
> — *Patricia Pealock, 52, Palmyra, NJ*

Seniors, as a rule, have more "time" to do with as they wish. However, so many seniors concern themselves with how little time is left and wonder where it went. No one, at any age, knows how much time is left. Therefore, it is wise to live each day to its fullest. Be grateful for the historic value of yesterday and make plans for tomorrow.
> — *Beverly T. Shedd, 71, Newmarket, NH*

To reach the age of ninety-plus, and I have, you must sleep if possible at least eight hours a night and in a well-ventilated room.
> — *Ted White, 90, Ramsey, NJ*

Take a trip. Order a wheelchair in advance if you need to change planes. Dress in a seasonal suit, silk hose, medium heels, white gloves and a becoming medium-brimmed hat. (Look regal: sit up straight... walk tall.) Tip well. You can go anywhere following this rule.
— *Doris R. Haddock, 86, Peterborough, NH*

The first thing to remember is that all your skills and abilities are only loaned to you for the short while that you are here on this earth. So make the most of them while you can.
— *Stephen J. Fraunberger, 79, Toms River, NJ (Died: Oct. 4, 1996)*

Don't be too rigid; a sip of dandelion wine on holidays won't hurt.
— *Inez Ross, 66, Los Alamos, NM*

Just as an oyster carries a pearl of great worth, it is the spirit within that matters.
— *Mary B. Bem, 70, Albuquerque, NM*

The main thing in life is to look forward, and not look back.
— *Josephine Degener, 100, Buffalo, NY*

At age 87, I still do it all (in moderation), except that last year I started rollerblading instead of ice skating (rollerblading has a longer season than ice skating)!
— *John Henry, 87, Wantagh, NY*

One of my most constant and satisfying pleasures is writing to a good friend. Try it, young people. It will help you through some rough times.
— *Elaine Lagerstrom, 72, Wilmington, NC*

When you face a loss of any kind—which is what aging involves—let the feelings surge and rise. Let the broken dreams and sadness speak. Do not shut your anger in and let it hurt your precious soul. Find a listener. There is hope in the midst of pain. Trust in the God who created you and is now shaping you for that new and creative second half of your life.
— *William E. Gramley, 60, Winston-Salem, NC*

Relationships enclose you in a "warm and fuzzy" atmosphere, helping you realize you are important to at least one other person. By retreating from people just because you're "old," you are defeating the real purpose of life—to give of yourself and the talents God entrusted only to you.
— *Arlene L. Isaak, 70, Arnegard, ND*

Don't ever stop asking "why?" You ask, "How did you get to be so old?" Now that is a good question. I think the reason is I have always wanted to learn why things are they way they are. So, please, keep right on asking, "Why?" If you don't you'll never, ever know.
— *Louis G. Haas, 88, Cornish Flat, NH*

You have only failed when you have failed to try. So, do your best and dream your future.
— *Rosemary Clary, 52, Laurelville, OH*

My wife and I have made it a priority to set aside time just for each other. This sounds simple, but unless one makes an effort, other commitments can creep in and time for nurturing one's primary relationship is too often sacrificed. During all our years of marriage, romance was part of our lives. We had dinner dates, sent special cards to say "I love you," and did small but meaningful kindnesses for each other. I believe this leads to Healthy Aging.
— *Donald H. Wood, 60, Cincinnati, OH*

Hang your dishrag in the sunshine and let the wind blow the laundry on the line. Examine a spider web. Breathe deeply of hyacinth, sweetpeas, and roses. Watch the sky on a clear night for a falling star. Enjoy nature's wonder.
— *Patricia C. Koehler, 71, Portland, OR*

Realize that, although you are one small person in the same boat with a lot of other people, you can find a way to paddle together.
— *Linda Burkett O'Hern, 51, Oklahoma City, OK*

I don't smoke and I don't drink. . . but I *do* cuss. . . I suppose that relives tension and stress. I try to learn something each day, as I know that when you are green you grow. . . when you are ripe. . . you rot!. . .And I don't want that!
— *Mary Lee Evans, 64, Tulsa, OK*

Eat a little, drink a little, and be merry and each day will be a new adventure. This is what Healthy Aging is all about.
— *Phyllis S. Angermann, 93 1/2, Philadelphia, PA*

Karate training has built character for many, even those over 50. Disciplines having noble grounding serve as a framework for living.
— *Robert C. Dilks, Sr., 63, Warren, PA*

Achieve a good mental outlook on life by reading novels and doing crossword puzzles. Join social organizations such as Lions Club, Elks, or church organizations.
— *Vincent De Pasquale, 73, Cranston, RI*

The most important ingredient in Healthy Aging is love—giving love and being able to recognize and receive love. Receiving love is sometimes difficult because it may be hard to recognize. Like the sun shining on your face, or a cool breeze on a hot afternoon. A dog chasing a ball and putting it at your feet. A cat curled up at the foot of your bed. A rainbow after a spring shower. Learn to look for ways to give and receive love.
— *Martha Chelena, 57, Myrtle Beach, SC*

Laugh at the wrinkles.
— *Constance R. Krueger, 50, Rapid City, SD*

Each individual needs to take responsibility to save and invest for the aging years from the first day of employment. Avoid using credit for instant gratification.
— *Frances C. Kauffman, 77, Memphis, TN*

Find at least two forms of exercise you thoroughly enjoy, one for summer, the other for winter.
— *Joann H. Gaffaney, 65, Rapid City, SD*

You'll live and grow if you never stop reading.
— *Sarah N. Wilson, 88, Oak Ridge, TN*

Reflections contribute to Healthy Aging. Thinking about what you have accomplished for those who will follow you, and what you would yet like to do, allows insight into both past and the future.
— *Jean Ehnebuske, 50, Georgetown, TX*

My advice for you when you retire, do not stop working. Former President Carter is building homes for the homeless. A hospital in our city has people working in it that retired years ago. Work in your village.
— *Alton S. Newell, 83, San Antonio, TX*

Be open to change. I grew up on an Indian Reservation. I rode in a wagon pulled by horses to get water for cooking. Fifty-six years later, I am writing to you on a computer! This miracle is a part of life and the existence we all share.
— *Roberta Windchief, 56, Neola, UT*

To cultivate a happy heart is really quite simple. . . Never spend more than ten minutes a day feeling sorry for yourself.
— *Janet Hayward Burnham, 59, Bethel, VT*

Accept change as a challenge. People who fear or reject change are like uprooted trees; they dry brittle and die bitter. Be a limber willow tree. Ask, how can I use change to my advantage? Remember, neither environment nor people control your thoughts nor your choices, only you can do that.
— *N. Elizabeth Bataineh, 62, Sterling, VA*

How I wish I had lived our lives "twice!" If I would have just slowed our lives down and at our Sunday meal have relived our week, we could all have learned more from our situations. Without constantly being on "fast-forward," just "pause" and reflect.
— *Mrs. Wally Geiger, 67, Troutville, VA*

If you are lucky enough to have a firm belief in some higher being, work at strengthening that faith. I think it is a form of life insurance after all. No matter how rotten the day may have been, never go to sleep without having a word with that higher being. Say a "Thank You" for the day. After all, it *was* another day.
— *Carmel Eitt, 79, King George, VA*

My children give me the impression that I'm capable of doing anything I've always done. That has given me the confidence and determination to live up to their expectations.
— *Kathleen N. Walker, 85, Clarksville, VA*

Lighten your load. Start now and avoid the estate sale later. Fill your home with only your absolutely most favorite things in the whole, wide world, and consign your surplus to charity.
— *Whitney I. Blair, 52, Newport News, VA*

Always remember that we get old outside but inside we have the same feelings, hopes, and beliefs as we did when we were young.

— *Alice M. Powell, 82, Kent WA*

I recommend that you keep a scrapbook. Fill it with your children's achievements and announcements and newspaper clippings and photos. You'll end up with a marvelous family history that will be enjoyed for generations.

— *Nona J. Eschbach, 66, Medina, WA*

Don't be afraid to re-examine your life when it ceases to be joyful. Take risks! If you must pack up and travel the solitary path to find the work, people, and places that allow you to live your deepest values. On life's journey there are bends in the road; welcome them. They will allow you to grow into the person you want to be.

— *Carole Nelson, 58, Seattle WA*

If you enjoy dancing—do it. Re-visit dance crazes of 1920s, 1950s.

— *Herbert Collins, 64, Washington, DC*

Don't live for tomorrow, live for now. The most important things don't cost money.

— *Jean Ramsey-Chefren, 52, Worthington, WV*

As I observe my dear 88-year-old mother walking to our rural mailbox to send a letter and then being so elated to receive a personal note, it makes me recognize the value of this endeavor.

— *Elaine, S. Fugate, 60, Triadelphia, WV*

The best advice I can give you is to start planning financially for your future *now*. Put the maximum amount allowed in your company's 401 or savings plan. It's the painless way to "pay yourself first."

— *Jim Jensen, 51, Portage, WI*

We don't sit on our children's doorsteps asking what they can do for us. It's refreshing what we can do for them.

— *Mrs. Etta Proeber, 68, Kenosha, WI*

The pathway to Healthy Aging lies in stretching. If life seems a little stiff in the morning, stretch it.

— *Mary Jean Lunne, 50, Gillette, WY*

Index